NATURE'S REMEDIES FOR STRESS AND FATIGUE

RECOVERING FROM BURNOUT

Jo Dunbar

WATKINS
1893

Nature's Remedies for Stress and Fatigue
Jo Dunbar

First published in the UK and USA 2024 by
Watkins, an imprint of Watkins Media Limited
Unit 11, Shepperton House, 89–93 Shepperton Road
London N1 3DF

enquiries@watkinspublishing.com

A CIP record for this book is available from
the British Library

ISBN: 978-1-78678-871-9 (paperback)
ISBN: 978-1-78678-873-3 (ebook)

1 3 5 7 9 10 8 6 4 2

Printed and bound by CPI Group (UK) Ltd, Croydon, CR0 4YY

www.watkinspublishing.com

Publisher's note:
The information in this book is not intended as a substitute for professional medical advice and treatment. If you are pregnant or breastfeeding or have any special dietary requirements or medical conditions, it is recommended that you consult a medical professional before following any of the information or recipes contained in this book. Watkins Media Limited, or any other persons who have been involved in working on this publication, cannot accept responsibility for any errors or omissions, inadvertent or not, that may be found in the recipes or text, nor for any problems that may arise as a result of preparing one of these recipes or following the advice contained in this work.

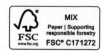

CONTENTS

PART 1
HOW STRESS AFFECTS YOUR BODY

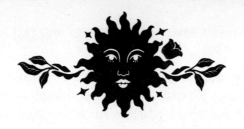

CHAPTER 1

WHAT IS CHRONIC FATIGUE?

This is a book about chronic fatigue – not the normal everyday tiredness that everyone has from time to time, but a deep, bone-aching exhaustion which is not alleviated by sleep, lasts for months or years, and affects almost every aspect of a person's life. This largely unrecognized syndrome is estimated to affect between 17 and 24 million people in the world, and the numbers are growing.

One of the reasons chronic fatigue is often unrecognized is that there is no definitive laboratory test to identify it. In our modern-day usage, "chronic" has taken on the meaning of "severe", but in medical parlance it actually means "ongoing, long-term or recurring". Additionally, the word "syndrome" refers to a group of symptoms which tend to occur together but have no identifiable cause, as opposed to a disease, which has clearly defined causation.

Without a visible wound or a blood test result to confirm diagnosis, the sufferer of long-term fatigue can feel as if their condition is not being taken seriously by others, who simply can't understand why they find day-to-day living so hard. Furthermore, without a basic understanding of why they are ill, there is no clear pathway to recovery.

This book aims to give you some understanding as to why you may feel so unwell, discussing several causes of chronic fatigue and what can be done to regain your robust health once again. Our understanding of this condition is incomplete, and no doubt more will be uncovered in the coming years, but I shall endeavour to tell you what the most recent research shows, and how to combat some of the main underlying causes based on my 25 years of experience helping people to recover from this illness using plant medicines and lifestyle changes.

A note on CFS/ME

I will not be writing specifically about chronic fatigue syndrome (CFS) or myalgic encephalomyelitis (ME), although what I discuss may very well be chronic fatigue syndrome or ME.

The problem is that, while there are several theories, no one can point to a clear, underlying cause for CFS or ME. There are lists of associated symptoms, but these are often interchangeable with other illnesses, such as Lyme disease, or a low thyroid state.

So, instead, I have chosen to write about what I believe are the major underlying causes of chronic fatigue syndrome/ ME, but instead of using this terminology, I will simply refer to the condition of "chronic fatigue".

Our over-busy lives

In my experience of treating CFS/ME, a significant number of cases develop out of the more extreme end of adrenal fatigue.* Also known as burnout or "TATT" (tired all the time), most of the patients I see are suffering from adrenal fatigue to some degree, although not everyone I see is

---

* Please note that adrenal fatigue is not the same as adrenal insufficiency, the extreme end of that being Addison's disease, which appears to be the only form of poor adrenal function that doctors recognize apart from tumours.

suffering from CFS/ME. Many are professional people, living ordinary lives, and yet feel as if they are dragging themselves around. They may experience recurrent chest infections from which they have difficulty recovering, have almost constant mouth ulcers, frequent cold sores, a bloated stomach, difficulty conceiving, and generally feel exhausted and debilitated.

When we are stressed, there is an over-stimulation of our central nervous system, which triggers the adrenal glands to release the hormones that help us deal with said stress. This is normal and entirely appropriate, except that in the current social environment within which we live, the stimulation is relentless, and our minds and bodies are becoming overwhelmed.

When I see people with chronic fatigue and ask them about their lives prior to the illness, there was always one or several "normal" life stressors which just went on and on. Whilst, unfortunately, it is rather normal to get used to these symptoms, we were not designed to live in this constant state of overload.

We were never meant to live like this.

After millions of years of evolution, during which we were very slowly adapting our habits, we finally evolved into *Homo sapiens* around 200,000 years ago. We lived in tribes, with a sense of community, mutual support, and accountability to the group. We were in tune with the natural rhythms of the earth, and moved at a human pace. Of course, living naturally had its stresses, but those were usually short and sharp – being attacked by a raiding party from another clan, for example, or having to deal with a hungry predator.

The stressful event would be dramatic, sometimes deadly, but it is not prolonged. The emergency passes and, if they're lucky, they live to tell the story to the other members of the tribe; they are not alone in their world. Their stress is recognized, shared and, importantly, is not a daily occurrence.

This is how we evolved to live over hundreds of thousands of years, then, suddenly, in the last few centuries, there was a dramatic acceleration in learning, industrialization and technology.

In our modern-day lives, typically we aren't being attacked on a daily basis by men with spears, and yet we are being subjected to almost continual low-grade alarms: to meet targets, to race back to the car to avoid a parking fine, to get the kids to school on time, to remember to pick up food for dinner. We are also silently dealing with the stresses of others not in our immediate vicinity, with images of wars and starvation on other continents filling our news feeds and drip-feeding terror into our subconsciousness. Coping with unrelenting stress is extremely energy-consuming. Small wonder that so many people are tired all the time.

From an evolutionary and biological perspective, our bodies are still entrenched in ancient patterns, and they're really struggling to keep up with our radically changed lifestyles. So, while our technology and brains are zooming ahead, our mental, emotional and physical bodies are strained to near breaking point. We no longer live at a "human" pace, and our bodies were never designed to live under such relentless stress.

Just like a rock subjected to pressure over time, eventually it will give way and break into pieces. Likewise, people can survive and function with chronic stress for years, and sometimes all it takes is one major or even seemingly minor life event to tip you into a long-term debilitating illness. Quite often, the internal cracks are not recognized until we actually collapse.

Fatigue is not depression

Before Long Covid, there was a predilection for treating unknown fatigue as depression, or worse. Having worked with chronic fatigue for many years, however, I have never met a patient who developed chronic fatigue because of depression. Instead, many developed some degree of depression *because* of chronic fatigue and the difficulties associated with living with this largely unrecognized illness.

Not only does chronic fatigue significantly impair your ability to earn a living, and to express yourself creatively, but in these high-cost-of-living days, you can imagine that spouses soon become dismayed at the diminished second income, and caring for their partner can also take its toll, mentally, emotionally and physically. This can make for dark days in the home, and as far as I can tell, the mainstream medical profession has nothing to offer the sufferer besides anti-depressants.

Complementary medicine tends to take a more holistic view, considering the mental, emotional, physical and, sometimes, spiritual aspects of a person's life. Medical herbs and nutritional supplements have actions that pharmaceutical drugs don't, and vice versa, so instead of an "us and them" approach, I believe they can work together, and that integrated medicine is the way forward. Sometimes, anti-depressants can give the patient the mental stability needed to even begin the work of recovery.

While I treat patients with chronic fatigue, I hold in mind that the body knows exactly what to do to heal itself. It is central to holistic medicine that we, the practitioners, simply provide the tools for the body to do what it does best – keep us alive. I also take comfort in the fact that herbs and humans have evolved together over the millenia. They know each other. Our bodies recognize the herbal constituents, and together they are far wiser than I can ever be. So, I provide the tools for the body, and the body does the repairing. My job is to try to work out which tools the body needs.

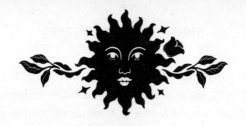

CHAPTER 2

THE PHYSIOLOGY OF STRESS

Stress is something we all feel from time to time, but when it is relentless, the body eventually buckles under the strain. In order to understand how stress affects the body, we need to look at the physiology of stress – what actually happens inside our cells when we become stressed. Once we understand this, we can have a much clearer idea of how to repair the damage.

When we register or anticipate a stressful situation, the brain immediately sends an urgent message of alarm to the sympathetic nervous system (SNS), which responds by instigating a series of physiological and hormonal changes in the body that will prepare it to face whatever threat is imminent. Within seconds of the alarm being raised, the SNS sends impulses to the adrenal glands, which immediately release stress hormones into the bloodstream.

One of these is adrenaline (also known as epinephrine), the body's short-term response to stress, which signals to the body to increase blood glucose levels, raise blood pressure and heart rate; dilate airways to raise oxygen levels; dilate blood vessels to enhance oxygenation of the muscles while constricting blood vessels to organs which are non-essential at the time of danger; and increasing mental alertness and shortening reaction times.

If, however, the stress is ongoing, then the stress response becomes mediated by the hormone cortisol. To prepare your body for long-term stress survival, cortisol will trigger the release of glucose for quick available energy; reduce inflammation, which helps recovery from injury; down-regulate the immune system; and constrict blood vessels, possibly to reduce blood loss in times of injury and to keep our blood pressure up so that we don't pass out.

When these hormones reach the brain, it responds by continuing to send the alarm messages to the SNS and the adrenal glands – thus a cycle of alarm continues until the person's brain perceives a reason to calm down.

This is what's called "fight or flight", or the acute stress response, and it is perfectly healthy and life-saving, but only for occasional, short periods of time.

Once the brain registers that the emergency is over, it sends a message of "all is well" to the nervous system by flicking over to the restful parasympathetic nervous system (PNS). Most of us live in a highly stressful world, which results in us secreting far more adrenaline and cortisol than we were ever meant to, and this can have a detrimental effect on our health. Moreover, with repeated or constant stress, the adrenal glands have to secrete adrenaline and cortisol on such a frequent basis that it barely gives any time for their recovery.

GAS and homeostasis

In the 1930s, Dr Hans Selye, an eminent endocrinologist from Hungary, coined the term "stress" to describe the body's reaction to alarm. He observed that whatever the cause of stress, our bodies will go to every necessary length to maintain homeostasis* within the cellular environment in order to preserve life, and that there was a predictable and

---

* *Homeo* – meaning "the same", and *stasis* – meaning "long period without change". So, homeostasis means "staying the same over an extended period of time".

observable pattern to this response, which Dr Selye called "general adaptation syndrome", or GAS.

Dr Selye divided the body's response to stress into three stages: alarm, resistance and exhaustion.

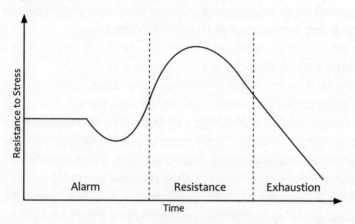

Stages of general adaptation syndrome

Stage 1: Alarm

Alarm is registered. The mind/body recognizes the danger and instantly prepares to survive with the "fight or flight" response. This is occurring at both a conscious and subconscious level in the brain and the cells. The internal environment is on high alert, but coping very well. You are "on it"!

This is the stage which our caveman ancestors experienced as surprise, fear and anger when, for example, their hunting party was attacked by a rival clan. If they survived the experience, they returned home knowing that they were once again safe. This stage is normally short-lived, and the homeostasis within the cells rapidly recovers, with little impact on short- or long-term health. These temporary periods of alarm are entirely normal and contribute to the excitement of life.

As we all know, however, our modern lives are very different to those of our ancestors. We experience these short-term shocks, albeit to a milder degree, at least several times a week, if not many times in a day. For the body to marshal these resources of survival, it is important to bear in mind that a great deal of energy is required.

Stage 2: Resistance

If the stressful situation has not been resolved, the body learns to adapt to this state of affairs. At this stage, there is no outward sign of danger to health, but the body is working so hard to maintain homeostasis that is not able to fully recover.

Because the adrenal glands produce higher-than-normal levels of cortisol, the immune system starts to flag, which means the body becomes more susceptible to infection. Sleep quality is poorer because of the raised cortisol, which means rest and recovery is less likely, and the adrenal glands become markedly fatigued.

"Every stress leaves an indelible scar, and the organism pays for its survival after a stressful situation by becoming a little older."
– Dr Hans Selye

It is quite likely that, in this stage, the person is completely unaware that they are struggling, or, more likely, they have learned not to take any notice. This is the point at which people often lean on caffeine and sugar for energy, and yet the stimulant effect of the caffeine flogs the adrenal glands even harder. The person's reserves are already at breaking point, and the caffeine, repeated alarm reaction and sugar stimulation push their resources to the brink.

Stage 3: Exhaustion

At some point, the person realizes they can no longer keep going, and that something is very wrong. To have reached this stage, the stress would have been prolonged and the effects of trying to survive have stacked up to unsustainable proportions. The body's resources have become just about depleted. The immune system is weak, and the adrenal glands are debilitated and not managing to maintain optimal cortisol levels. The person is unable to resist or cope with stress.

By this stage, we would say the person has "hit the wall". They feel exhausted, irritable, depressed and tearful, are unable to fight off minor infections such as colds, and so become repeatedly ill. Recovery from these illnesses also takes longer each time. Their muscles may be painful and they are unable to think clearly.

This is what is commonly called adrenal fatigue syndrome. It does not describe normal, run-of-the-mill fatigue, and demands a lifestyle change.

Adrenal fatigue symptom checklist

Adrenal hormonal levels can be checked using private laboratory tests, which are usually arranged by a health practitioner, but this symptom checklist is a good start.

Have a look the following lists of symptoms and check those that apply to you.

If you find you have ticked several symptoms, especially at least one in each category, there is a possibility that you may be suffering from adrenal fatigue.

Sleeping and waking

☐ I have difficulty getting out of bed in the morning.

☐ I often don't feel fully awake for hours.

☐ I wake up feeling as tired as I did when I went to bed.

☐ I have difficulty falling asleep at night.

☐ I feel tired all day, but suddenly feel wide awake and wonderful after 11 p.m.

☐ I fall asleep but wake frequently during the night.

Mental and emotional

☐ My brain feels foggy and I cannot concentrate on what I am doing.

☐ I have difficulty staying focused on conversations.

☐ I feel extra sensitive to noise and light.

☐ I frequently have headaches.

☐ I cannot cope with any stress. I either want to hide or I become very intolerant.

☐ I feel as if I want to avoid people, even friends. I just want to be alone.

☐ I can feel tearful for no reason.

☐ I can't cope anymore.

☐ I am not ill because I am depressed. I am depressed because I am ill.

☐ I have irrational flashes of anger which I know are unreasonable, but I can't seem to help myself.

Physical

☐ I feel bone-achingly tired all the time. This is not a normal tiredness.

☐ Everything I do takes so much effort.

☐ My mind is willing, but my body just won't do it.

☐ My muscles ache.

☐ My muscles feel very weak and tender.

☐ Wounds take a long time to heal.

☐ I cannot regulate my temperature.

☐ I urinate a lot.

☐ I feel shaky inside.

☐ I feel cold or tender over the kidney area in my back.

☐ If I do anything, it can take an extraordinary amount of time to recover.

Reproduction

☐ I have lost my sex drive.

☐ My pre-menstrual symptoms have got worse.

☐ I cannot conceive.

Food and digestion

☐ I often crave sugar, salt or caffeine.

☐ I can wake in the night with a terrible thirst or hunger.

☐ I regularly get the feeling that I just HAVE to eat.

☐ My stomach frequently feels bloated and gassy.

☐ My food remains undigested – like a brick in my stomach.

☐ I often feel nauseous.

Immune system

☐ I have never quite recovered from a viral infection.

☐ I get colds all the time and find it difficult to recover.

☐ I never get ill; I just never feel well.

☐ I have frequent mouth ulcers or cold sores.

☐ I often have swollen glands in my neck.

☐ I have developed multiple allergies.

☐ I frequently have a sore throat.

Circulatory system

☐ I am often dizzy when I stand up.

☐ I have heart palpitations, even when resting.

☐ My limbs are often very cold.

☐ I often have blue legs.

When I treat chronic fatigue, I will always treat the adrenal glands, as well as the nervous system, the immune system and, highly likely, the reproductive, thyroid and digestive systems, too. Before we move onto what you can do about this disease, let us look at the effects that stress has on the health of some of our body systems.

How stress makes us ill

Our understanding of the effects of stress on our physiology is still pretty rudimentary. However, by simply looking at the effects of one stress hormone – cortisol – and the over-stimulation of the nervous system, we can start to see just how devastating the effects of stress can be to our health and wellbeing.

Stress affects the adrenal glands

As Hans Selye outlined in the early part of the last century, when stress hits us, we tend to be knocked off course for a short period. At that time, the adrenal glands secrete lots of adrenaline and cortisol, which helps us to cope with the situation. The immune system is in fact stimulated, and very soon we gather ourselves together and get on with our lives.

However, as we've seen, if the stress becomes prolonged, the adrenal glands are compelled to continue secreting cortisol and adrenaline. After some time, the glands become fatigued. They cannot maintain this level of high alert.

Once fatigued, the adrenal glands will produce less and less cortisol. At this point the person feels that they cannot cope with any more stress, and this is because they are right: their body *physiologically* can no longer cope with the stress. If the stress persists, the adrenal glands valiantly oblige by secreting what little cortisol they are able to manufacture. Eventually, the person develops adrenal fatigue, also known as adrenal exhaustion, burnout, or what was once called neurasthenia. This condition is characterized by body pain, mental and physical exhaustion, a feeling of brain fog and a strong aversion to stimuli or stress of any kind, among other symptoms.

Healthy adrenal glands will secrete a sharp peak of cortisol within half an hour of waking in the morning. This should give us the "get up and go" that we need for the day ahead. The levels of cortisol drift down during the day, so that they are very low in the evening when we prepare for bed and rest. If you measure the cortisol levels of severely fatigued people, there is a blunted or very little no peak.

Another adrenal hormone called aldosterone keeps our fluid levels in balance by controlling the sodium and potassium balance. Aldosterone is the anti-diuretic hormone – in other words, it holds the fluid in our bodies. With adrenal fatigue, this hormone may also become difficult to produce, and many people find themselves urinating frequently, often a pale and copious urine, and may develop a great thirst and craving for salty food. It is likely that the salt serves the purpose of holding water in the body when aldosterone is low.

In my practice I see people with this condition every day, and it is my opinion that adrenal fatigue can be a major forerunner to full-scale chronic fatigue syndrome.

Some studies suggest that chronic fatigue syndrome shows "staggering similarities to Addison's disease",[1] which is complete adrenal failure. In 1998, scientists used a CT scan to measure the size of the adrenal glands in a group of people with chronic fatigue syndrome. In each case, the glands had shrunk by over 50%, "indicating significant adrenal atrophy in Chronic Fatigue Syndrome patients".[2] Interestingly, liquorice is the old-fashioned treatment for Addison's disease, and this is one of the best herbs to help restore the adrenal glands, and a major herb to use in the recovery from CFS.

Stress affects the blood sugar levels

When the brain registers alarm, it sends an emergency message to the adrenal glands telling them to release adrenaline and cortisol so that the body can spring into action and effectively deal with the object of alarm. This potentially life-saving burst of energy requires immediate fuel, and therefore an instant supply of blood sugar is needed, whether the person has recently eaten or not.

Cortisol helps to maintain homeostasis by lifting the levels of glucose in the blood when blood sugars are dipping. Glucose is the most available source of energy in the blood; and in the liver, cortisol converts amino acids (derived from protein) into glucose. From there, the glucose passes into the blood where it is sent to the muscles and brain to use as energy.

The body relies on cortisol to top up the blood sugar levels between meals and during periods of starvation when blood sugar has dropped. In a healthy person, cortisol maintains balanced blood sugar levels during periods of stress or fasting, thus preventing hypoglycaemia. However, if the adrenal glands have become fatigued, and still the body requires a sudden rise in blood sugar levels, the cortisol is not present in sufficient quantities to perform this task.

One of the most obvious signs of fatigued adrenal glands is when the person experiences sudden sugar cravings, because their adrenal glands are no longer able to maintain their blood sugar levels effectively. Perhaps you have experienced this yourself when you feel that you need to eat a sugary snack *right now*, and can become quite agitated or even aggressive if your blood sugar levels drop too much. The term often used is "hangry" (hungry and angry). The sugar is actually supplementing your body's ability to supply the necessary glucose itself. Now, once you have eaten the sugar, your blood sugar levels shoot up, and you feel wonderful again – for a short while.

When a person eats a sugary snack, within minutes the sugar levels in the blood are elevated to a peak, and the pancreas has to quickly release insulin to bring the sugar levels down to balance again. But insulin is not a precise hormone, and the blood sugar tends to plummet to a very low level again – thus, sooner or later, the person needs more sugar to push the blood sugars back up. Many people live like this, with their blood sugar levels soaring and plummeting throughout the day, and you can imagine that this is very stressful for the body, which is constantly trying to maintain a homeostatic balance. This type of lifestyle cannot be sustained in the long term, and ultimately something will have to give. If that person does not change towards a more sustainable way of living, then it will be their health that gives way, in the end.

It is often stated that cortisol and insulin work in opposition to each other, and in a narrow sense that is correct. It is the job of cortisol to increase blood glucose, while it is the job of insulin to pack away the glucose into the cells, thus reducing blood sugar levels. However, the reality is that they try to work together to ensure that the levels of glucose in the bloodstream are kept within a narrow healthy range.

It is the norm in our society for people to live highly stressful lives, and consequently also have elevated cortisol levels. This means that they probably also have elevated blood sugar levels, and thus elevated insulin levels, and insulin resistance which can lead to Type 2 diabetes, cardiovascular disease, obesity, abnormal cholesterol levels or polycystic ovary syndrome.

Insulin resistance can also affect the central nervous system. Although the brain accounts for only 2% of our body weight, it requires 20–30% of blood glucose for clear cognitive functioning. With insulin resistance, the cells in the brain cannot get hold of the glucose required to think clearly, and this condition has been linked to cognitive dysfunction (brain fog).[3]

Yeast overgrowth is another common outcome that occurs when tired people use sugary snacks and caffeine to keep themselves going. The high levels of sugar feeds yeast cells, such as the *Candida albicans*, among others, which live in our intestines. We all know from school biology that yeast thrives in a dark, moist and sugary environment, so when your immune system is exhausted, and you are feeding the yeast in your gut with lots of sugar – there is nothing to hold the yeast population back from exploding.

Candida overgrowth is another unrecognized condition by the medical establishment, unless the person is immuno-suppressed with cancer, AIDS or organ transplant, etc., but nutritionists and other complementary therapists deal with *Candida* all the time.

A *Candida* overgrowth in the gut can penetrate the intestinal wall with root-like hyphae into the bloodstream, often overwhelming the immune system.[4] Systemic candidiasis can produce many symptoms which are very similar to adrenal fatigue, such as brain fog, muscle pain and lethargy, and it is not uncommon for people to suffer from both candidiasis and adrenal fatigue.

Stress affects our waistline

You might think that high stress and high cortisol means that fat and protein are going to be burned extra hard for fuel, and you are bound to lose lots of weight. Annoyingly not. On the contrary, cortisol stimulates your desire for high-sugar, high-fat foods.

If you think about it, it is quite logical. You might have evolved to live in a sophisticated city, but your body still thinks that it is living in the savannah. As far as it is concerned, any stress might as well be a charging lioness, and that means that it needs to run fast. To get you out of the situation as quickly as possible, instant glucose is required. The elevated cortisol stimulates the intense desire to eat highly calorific foods, which can be used to save you from the ever-present lioness.

Elevated cortisol levels are well known to cause belly fat, and people who take steroid medication over a period of time develop round, fatty waistlines and thin arms and legs. This is what happens in the body when we are over-exposed to natural cortisol – fat is deposited around the belly and the organs of the abdomen.

Stress affects our thyroid gland

The thyroid gland is located at the front of our throat, and you might think of it as the thermostat of the body, as it regulates the body temperature and metabolic rate. If your thyroid function is under-active, you feel sluggish, cold, fatigued all the time, and you gain weight despite eating very little. Constipation is common, and hair and skin can become coarse, whilst the outer edges of eyebrows thin. You may also experience brain fog, feel mentally sluggish and depressed.

You might have noticed that some of the symptoms associated with a hypoactive thyroid are similar to those of adrenal fatigue. Although these are two separate conditions, it can happen that those who suffer from a low thyroid function not caused by an autoimmune disease may also suffer from poor adrenal function. To remedy the low thyroid function, you first need to restore the adrenal glands. I shall elaborate on this soon, but to understand how the two are linked, I need to explain a few things first.

In a healthy person, the pituitary gland in the brain secretes thyroid-stimulating hormone (TSH), which stimulates the thyroid gland to produce the inactive thyroid hormone T4. This is converted into the activated thyroid hormone T3 in the liver and kidneys, then enters the cells of the body, influencing metabolism.

Now, as you know, long-term stress can result in adrenal fatigue, and the body will always do whatever is required to survive. Whereas in the past, the person might have felt tired, but would not stop, now the body takes matters in hand and forces the person to rest by reducing the hormones which govern our energy. The body insists on regulating its own internal environment in order to improve the chances of survival, and we see this with elevated cortisol blood levels suppressing TSH as well as T3. When there is excessive cortisol in the blood, the pituitary gland's secretion of TSH and the thyroid gland's secretion of T4 can be down-regulated.[5] Cortisol can also inhibit the conversion of the inactive T4 into the active T3. Further down-regulation of thyroid activity can occur when T4 is not converted into active T3, but rather into reverse T3 (rT3). Reverse T3 is inactive and may even oppose the active T3.

Furthermore, cortisol can affect the availability of thyroid hormones to the cells. In order for these hormones to take effect in the body, they need to be freely circulating so that they can enter the cells and exert their effects. Thyroid hormones are carried around the blood, bound to thyroid-binding globulin (TBG). Stress may increase the activity of

TBG so that the thyroid hormones are unable to enter the cell. Like a key which is too large for the lock.

When someone presents me with the above symptoms, I will invariably check the adrenal function as well as the thyroid function. Some practitioners advocate only treating the adrenal glands on the basis that the thyroid will recover as the adrenal glands recover. I tend to focus my attention on the adrenal glands, but I do also give herbs and nutritional support to the thyroid gland (more on which later).

Stress affects our immune system

There is a lot of information available informing us how acute and chronic stress affects the immune system. Much of this information is the result of a relatively new science called psycho-neuro-endocrine-immunology (PNEI). This body of science takes as holistic an approach as is possible currently within mainstream science, attempting to look at how stress affects the whole body, and it is greatly improving our understanding of how the mind can cause physical illness, and why stress is so destructive to our health.

Like the rest of our body, the immune system is incredibly complicated and made up of several "departments". For the moment we shall concentrate on part of the immune system called the T-cells. These cells are manufactured in the thymus gland – hence the "T" in their name. There are several types of T-cells, but the ones we are going to focus on are called T-helper cells (Th cells). T-helper cells are divided into Th1 and Th2, which, like cortisol and insulin, work in opposition to each other – thus modulating each other.

Think of them like a pair of scales, with Th1 at one end and Th2 at the other. The balance of the scales swings equally between the two, with Th1 raised (dominating) from mid-morning to early evening, and Th2 raised (dominating) during the night and early morning. However, under some conditions, the body will be driven to be more permanently dominated by either a Th1 or Th2 response.

Th1 cells are geared towards killing viruses, bacteria and cancer cells.[6] The Th1 response gives us the typical symptoms of illness, such as fever, inflammation, malaise, loss of appetite, and withdrawal from society. You can understand now why we experience our cold and flu symptoms more in the evenings.

Th2 stimulates immunoglobulin E (IgE) and mast cells, which secrete histamine. Thus we see that when the immune system is in a state of Th2 domination, there is a greater propensity towards allergies, some autoimmune conditions, and post-viral fatigue (CFS/ME).[7]

During periods of short-term stress, the immune system swings into Th1 domination. This is what Hans Selye was observing when he described how the body rallies during a stressful event. This is the resistance part of the GAS model, where the immune system is actually stimulated, and thus you may have a cold and experience the usual symptoms such as fever and feeling generally unwell, but you quickly recover. If the stress is ongoing, the immune scales will then tip from Th1 to Th2 domination, and get stuck there.[8] It's a bit like the wheels of a car revving in the mud, putting in a lot of effort but getting nowhere. Over time the immune system becomes more and more exhausted, and now the person is less able to recover from viral illness (low Th1), and more prone to developing allergic or inflammatory conditions (high Th2).

Studies are starting to show that people suffering from chronic fatigue syndrome have a bias towards higher Th2 and lower Th1,[9] which means that they have higher prevalence to allergies and lower resistance to viruses. It is at this point, when many sufferers of chronic fatigue believe they got ill, but you can see that, actually, they have been gearing up for this illness for years.

It is not only chronic stress which shifts towards the Th2 domination, but also sleep deprivation (caused by high cortisol levels) and increased sympathetic nervous system activity – fight or flight (caused by stress and anxiety). Once this shift has occurred, it is not very easy to bring it back into balance.

We know that cortisol powerfully down-regulates the immune system. It is so powerful that a synthesized version of cortisol (cortisone) is used on patients with organ transplants to suppress the immune system so that the body won't reject the new organ. On the one hand, cortisol is anti-inflammatory, which is absolutely necessary for survival in the case of injury, but this is only useful in the short term. Long-term elevated levels of cortisol massively reduce the immune system's ability to adequately respond to bacteria, fungi and viruses.

Over time, sufferers of chronic fatigue have such depleted immune systems that they just cannot fight off viruses or fungi any longer. To fight the viruses, they need the Th1 response, which will raise the body temperature. Many invading organisms can only survive in a very narrow temperature band and raising the body temperature can be enough to kill them. However, for the body to raise its temperature by even 1°C, it takes over 10% of our available energy,[10] and, as well as being stuck in Th2 domination, these people simply do not have the energy resources to achieve the temperature rise.

This is why the correct herbal medicine and diet are absolutely fundamental to recovery, and why, after some months of work, when my CFS patients tell me that they have had a cold – we celebrate. The immune system has "clicked back" into balance and recovery can begin.

Stress is related to inflammation and allergies

As we saw above, stress tips the immune scales towards the Th2 bias, which increases sensitivity to developing allergies. Many studies confirm the relationship between chronic stress and atopic reactions, e.g. asthma, eczema and hayfever, as well as increased allergies to foods. An allergy is an inappropriately high immune reaction to allergens such as pollen or food, leading to cells in the blood releasing inflammatory substances which irritate the mucous membranes. However, with fatigued adrenal glands unable to produce the cortisol which damps down the excessive immune response, the Th2 reaction is unopposed, and this may be one of the contributing factors to the increasingly high numbers of allergy sufferers we are seeing these days.

Stress is associated with inflammation in many parts of the body. In Romania, a group of 118 seemingly healthy physicians were studied, and the conclusion reached was that professional stress is connected with inflammation in the body, which might be responsible for cardiac disease.[11]

This was supported by another study, which found raised inflammatory markers in the blood of a sample group of over 12,000 people who were suffering with anxiety and acute stress.[12]

One fascinating study described how stress-related cortisol disrupts the barrier of the intestine, promoting inflammatory bowel disease, and irritable bowel syndromes. Here the scientists describe the two-way communication known as the gut–brain axis. The mental stress stimulates the raised cortisol, which triggers mast cells to release histamine. The histamine in the gut causes the intestinal lining to become inflamed and permeable. They found that stress also caused dysbiosis, which is where there is too much of the unfriendly and not enough of the friendly bacteria. Stress resulted in reduced populations of the friendly *Lactobacillus* bacteria, allowing the opportunistic growth of unfriendly bacteria to grow.[13]

Stress even affects rheumatoid arthritis, where long-term stress stimulates Interleukin-6, a highly inflammatory substance, which triggers arthritic inflammation, pain and fatigue.[14]

There are so many studies linking stress to inflammation, illness and fatigue. The list above is only a tiny sample to give you an inkling of the havoc stress can wreak on your health and wellbeing.

Stress affects our brain function

We all know that serotonin is our "happy hormone", and is needed for appetite regulation and to keep us cheerful. However, less well known is that it is also related to body temperature regulation. Many of my chronic fatigue patients describe how they struggle with temperature regulation and tell me how they feel the cold far more acutely than their family. The part of the brain which regulates our temperature is in the hypothalamus. Long-term stress interrupts the serotonin interaction with this part of the brain, disrupting the healthy daily pattern of temperature regulation.[15]

It is one of the horrible ironies that people who are chronically fatigued frequently have difficulty falling asleep or staying asleep. Sleep, which used to come easily, is now elusive, and, of course, we all need sleep in order for our bodies to heal and restore equilibrium. Melatonin is a sleep hormone derived from serotonin, but if your cortisol levels are high, your serotonin levels will be low, and thus there will be less serotonin available to convert into melatonin. This translates into poor sleep and a disturbed night, which can be compounded if your adrenal glands are so fatigued that they are unable to produce the morning spike of cortisol necessary for you to wake bright-eyed in the morning. So, you might crash out the night before, but you will wake in the morning feeling as tired as you did when you went to bed.

The Montclair Memory Clinic in New York explains how ongoing stress can make it difficult to process, store and recall information due to the fact that long-term stress with raised levels of cortisol inhibits the production of new nerves cells in the brain to the point of shrinking your brain. Moreover, stress weakens the protective blood–brain barrier, allowing free radicals to infiltrate into the brain, further harming the nerve cells.

Prolonged elevated adrenal hormones can also directly affect memory and emotion by shrinking the hippocampus. This part of the brain is responsible for the formation of new memories and is associated with our emotional response. It is rich in receptors for cortisol, but if too many cortisol molecules dock into these receptors, they start to destroy the nerves, resulting in memory loss, poor concentration and difficulty learning.[16]

Over the years, I have noticed that of those people who have experienced chronic stress, and who show low cortisol levels in their test results, can become hyper-sensitive and even quite hostile in order to protect themselves from the stress which they know that they can no longer cope with. When upsetting or startling stresses occur, someone with burnout finds that they may lash out, or may startle very easily. They may feel anxious but without a reason, and experience difficulty recovering from general stresses of life. Any stress at all "knocks them for six" and they can take days to recover. No wonder they overreact to the smallest stress – they know that they simply do not have the resources to cope anymore.

This is why I believe it is so important to really understand why a person is depressed, and why I don't always prescribe St John's wort for depression. A person's depression, when understood in its full context after a proper consultation with the patient, will often show to be the result of stress (or despair) and may be linked with a thyroid, serotonin, cortisol or sex hormone imbalance. All of these issues need to be taken into account when treating a patient as a unique individual deserving of a unique approach to their illness.

Stress affects our reproductive system

There are so many women these days who suffer from poly-cystic ovary syndrome, infertility, pre-menstrual syndrome, fibroids, lumpy breasts or pre-menstrual water retention. What could possibly be going on?

An analysis of 42 studies of women with polycystic ovary syndrome showed that the cortisol levels in these women were significantly higher than those of healthy women.[17] Women who experience pre-menstrual tension have altered cortisol levels. Women who are exposed to increased stress and extended periods of elevated cortisol are 2.7 times more likely to miscarry,[18] and according to the Phoenix sperm bank, the normal paces and pressure of modern living can cause enough psychological stress to decrease testosterone, sperm count and motility with increased abnormal sperm production.

Both men and women who have lived with stress for so long that their cortisol levels are flagging are usually simply too tired to think about sex, while high stress and high cortisol levels in men can significantly inhibit the ability to achieve and maintain an erection.

A reason for this is that cortisol is a hormone necessary for survival of the individual, while the sex hormones are necessary for the survival of the race. In times of high stress (for instance when fleeing as a war-time refugee), the body prioritizes survival over reproduction, and will use the sex hormones to supplement cortisol in order to ensure that the individual survives. This is why some women stop menstruating when they are in a drastic situation. The same occurs to some women on long expeditions, or highly competitive athletes – the body cannot distinguish between fun stress and deadly stress.

In women, most of our progesterone is manufactured in the ovaries, but a small proportion is manufactured in the adrenal glands. When we are under prolonged stress and the adrenal glands are struggling to keep up with the demand for cortisol, an energy-saving mechanism for the adrenal glands is to steal ready-made progesterone from the ovaries and convert it into cortisol. This short-cut saves several steps in the conversion of cholesterol to cortisol, and provides the cortisol necessary for survival. This is known as the "progesterone steal". It is a bit like eating into your capital when money is tight – it saves the day, but ultimately it undermines your financial stability.

As a result, although there is now enough cortisol to cope with the stress, the progesterone levels start to become depleted. As the female progesterone levels drop, the correct ratio between oestrogen and progesterone becomes unbalanced, with oestrogen levels being higher than progesterone. As you have seen with other hormones, there is a natural check-and-balance system in our body. Oestrogen and progesterone naturally oppose and balance each other's effects. With the lowered progesterone levels, oestrogen becomes the dominant hormone. This is not the only reason why oestrogen may dominate progesterone, but it is a very important one.

Sub-optimal progesterone
Have a look at the following symptoms of sub-optimal progesterone and see if they relate to you:

- Pre-menstrual syndrome

- Fibromyalgia

- Short-term memory impairment

- Spasms and cramps

- Irritability

- Anxiety and/or depression

- Mood swings

- Difficulty sleeping

- Early miscarriage or difficulty conceiving

- Osteoporosis

- Joint pain.

The internet will tell you that if you have oestrogen dominance, you need to clear it with DIM (Diindolylmethane), and if you are low in progesterone, that you need to use progesterone cream. Hopefully, you realize now that these may not be long-term solutions, although they can be useful in the short term.

These days it is common for women to delay pregnancy until their late thirties or early forties, and by then so many feel "wired and tired" from very busy lifestyles and hectic work schedules, that it can be difficult for them to fall pregnant. I have found that if herbs and nutrition are used to support the adrenal glands, these women who previously could not conceive can often achieve a successful pregnancy.

In men, most of the testosterone comes from the testes, but some of the hormone is manufactured in the adrenal glands. In a man's mid-forties, testosterone will naturally start to decline, which is why men tend to mellow in their middle years. The adrenal glands will pick up the slack and contribute some testosterone, but if a man has been under tremendous stress and his adrenal glands are very fatigued, he literally becomes "knackered". The body will produce cortisol at the expense of testosterone.

Symptoms of sub-optimal testosterone

- Lack of joie de vivre

- Depression

- Increased irritability

- Difficulty concentrating

- Fatigue

- Little or no interest in sex

- Difficulty attaining or maintaining an erection

- Diminished muscle bulk and physical strength.

Stress affects our digestive system

The involuntary (autonomic) nervous system is divided into the sympathetic nervous system (fight or flight) and the parasympathetic nervous system (rest and digest), and these two systems have a profound effect on our digestion. When we are relaxed, our parasympathetic nervous system dominates and digestive enzymes are easily secreted. The peristaltic movements of the gut move in a coordinated wave-like motion so that we digest and absorb our food easily, and our bowels pass well-formed stools regularly.

When we feel anxious, the autonomic nervous system flicks like a switch from the parasympathetic nervous system (rest and digest) into the sympathetic nervous system mode of "flight or fight" as it prepares to cope with the situation. The blood supply is diverted away from the central areas of the body like the digestive tract and the digestive enzymatic secretions are switched off, while the muscles in the gut crunch up. There is wisdom in old-fashioned table manners where it is considered bad manners to discuss religion or politics at the dining table, because it is highly likely that an argument will ensue, which will interfere with digestion and the appreciation of the food on the table.

When we eat in a hurry or under stress, our parasympathetic nervous system is switched off and we do not secrete the digestive enzymes as we should do. Without adequate hydrochloric acid and digestive enzymes, the food cannot be broken down properly and it sits there like a brick in your stomach. Eventually it starts to ferment, producing gas, a feeling of bloating, flatulence and burping. The "anxious gut" seizes up, and the food is not moved along; instead the fermenting food produces toxins which in time can overburden the liver and inflame the gut lining, leading to a leaky gut.

Insufficient stomach acid fails to kill unfriendly bacteria which have been swallowed with the meal, and now these are able to multiply in our intestines, producing very smelly gas, and displacing our friendly bacteria – a process called dysbiosis. These unfriendly bacteria secrete toxins which also inflame the lining of the intestine, exacerbating the leakiness of the intestine walls, so that undigested food particles are able to slip through these holes into the bloodstream. This is how food intolerances begin, and this condition commonly manifests as symptoms such as joint pain, brain fog and lethargy, and, at the more extreme end, may trigger autoimmune conditions such as rheumatoid arthritis.

If you live with ongoing anxiety, it may be the norm that you experience painful stomach spasms which will probably be diagnosed as irritable bowel syndrome. The cramps and spasms are uncoordinated, interrupting the normal peristaltic movement of the bowels. Faecal matter in the bowel is not adequately evacuated, and the bowel becomes clogged. Toxins from old faecal matter seep back into the bloodstream through the lining of the colon, literally poisoning your system and over-burdening your liver. At the very least, you will have bad breath, but possibly your intestinal lining will become inflamed so that you cannot adequately absorb your nutrients.

All this is quite shocking, but it's only the tip of the iceberg. Long-term stress significantly affects every part of our bodies, and, alas, many of these illnesses are treated symptomatically and in isolation, and so the person remains ill for years because, sooner or later, another "illness" will emerge.

When a person is treated holistically, the practitionaer has an opportunity to get to know the client, and treat the whole person – certainly the mental, emotional and physical, and, if the person would like, then the spiritual aspect can be explored too. It goes beyond that; one must consider the person's lifestyle and diet, and sometimes be a listening ear for stories that cannot be told to anyone else.

A long-term solution may be to calm the person, discuss ways of slowing down their lifestyle, restoring optimal adrenal function, addressing the diet and particularly blood sugar stability and nutrition. Then, to treat the hormonal imbalances and symptoms, possibly discussing work–life balance or how to work and live in a way that is sustainable for the person for years to come, because we are all going to have to keep working for much longer than our parents had to. The sustainable solution to optimal wellness is to learn to live well. Sustainability is the name of the game, and we are learning that with the natural environment, with farming, heating and eating, and now we need to learn that we have to live sustainably too.

I propose that stress might be the greatest unacknowledged malady in our time. We must try to address the root of our dis-ease and do everything in our power to live more peacefully and in wellness. I am hopeful that we might learn to be kinder to ourselves and other Earth beings, so that we can thrive and live happily with robust health.

PART 2
HOW TO HELP
YOURSELF RECOVER

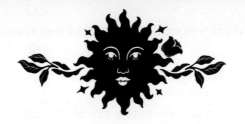

CHAPTER 3

BALANCING YOUR BLOOD SUGAR

Taking control of your diet and blood sugar levels will have an immediate and profound effect on your feeling of sturdiness. This is something that is completely in your control and the first step towards regaining your strength.

When your health has failed to the degree that you feel too exhausted to work efficiently (or at all), you can't bear the thought of interacting with friends and your body is in constant pain and you feel jittery and utterly fragile, one of the quickest things you can do to help yourself is to stabilize your blood sugar levels,

I frequently find that as people start to become aware of their increasing exhaustion, they fuel their lives with coffee and sugar. Gone are the days of a lunch hour. Now, instead of sitting down to eat decently, our modern culture demands that we eat at the desk, or on the run. This is completely insensible when you consider that the body cannot physiologically digest and absorb nutrients effectively in a state of heightened stimulation. Moreover, people are so over busy that they miss meals, allowing their blood sugar levels to crash, which inevitably means that soon enough they are desperate for a sugary snack to lift the blood sugars. Living like this is extremely common, and results in the blood sugars soaring and crashing like a ship in stormy waters, which is incredibly stressful on the body and unsustainable in the long term.

Too tired to digest

Your body uses approximately 10% of the calories that you eat to digest and absorb the nutrients, but that figure is a bit misleading, because protein digestion requires 20–30% of the total calories eaten. That is a lot of energy. Some of the people I have worked with are literally too fatigued to marshal the energy to digest their food, and so I advise my chronic fatigue patients to have six small, nutrient-dense meals a day.

The point is that when you are so very tired, you just don't have the energy to digest a large meal. It is much easier for the body to digest a small one.

Rebalancing blood sugar

Intermittent fasting is all the rage now, but this is not a helpful option for those with adrenal fatigue or burnout. One of the major symptoms that I have noticed in people suffering with long-term fatigue is that their blood sugars easily plummet, leaving them feeling weak, shaky and irritable. Unlike healthy people, the bodies of chronically fatigued people seem unable to efficiently raise their blood sugars without the help of food. Until your adrenal glands are restored, you will have to take care of your blood sugars by eating little and often through the day. Why, you may ask, is this so important?

If you are suffering from adrenal fatigue, rebalancing your blood sugars is absolutely fundamental to your recovery. The body considers low blood sugar levels to be a famine emergency and has to release more cortisol to turn proteins into glucose in order to raise the blood sugars again. But in order to recover, you need to take as much pressure off the adrenal glands as possible by providing small quantities of high-quality foods which provide slow-release energy to support the body. In this way, you send a message to the body that life is safe and secure, there is enough food, and the adrenals are not placed under any further stress.

This is not to say that you should eat sugary foods – they will just put you back on the sugar rollercoaster again, exhausting your pancreas and predisposing you to Type 2 diabetes. Don't deny yourself a little treat, but if you are going to have a sweet treat, have it after a meal, and don't overdo it.

Small quantities of highly nutritious foods will support your health. So, as little stress as possible and nice even blood sugar levels are the order of the day.

From the very first day that you begin to take care of your diet, you will feel the benefits. When your blood sugar levels become stabilized, you will feel as if you are living on much more solid ground. That jittery, hopeless, nearly hysterical feeling will instantly diminish, and the body will welcome proper food with high nutritional value.

Small, highly nutritious and more frequent meals are easy to digest, keep the blood sugars stable and nourish the cells with the nutrients that they need to recover health.

Please do avoid all caffeinated drinks, sugary snacks, and drastically reduce refined carbohydrates. Try to stay away from highly preserved foods, take-away junk food, and make all possible efforts to eat in a peaceful and convivial environment.

Don't forget what that wise old man Hippocrates said: "Let food be your medicine and medicine be your food."

If you are upset, your sympathetic nervous system will take over, diverting the blood away from the digestive tract, and shutting off the digestive enzymes. It's not a good scenario. When you stay calm, the parasympathetic nervous system dominates, so that your digestive enzymes flow, allowing for proper digestion and absorption of nutrients, thus feeding your body and your health.

Rest and digest.

Meal Suggestions

Breakfast

- Poached eggs on rye or spelt bread toast

- Sautéed mushrooms on rye or spelt bread toast

- Grilled goat's cheese on a bed of wilted spinach with a poached egg

- Tomato and fresh herb omelette

- Porridge oats with a sprinkle of cinnamon powder and half a grated apple, topped with sunflower and sesame seeds to provide some protein and good fats

- Avocado on wholegrain toast with lime juice. Add some smoked salmon or smoked tofu if it appeals.

- A small bowl of live plain yoghurt, with plenty of fresh fruit, nuts and seeds

- Slices of tomatoes with raw onions and olive oil on toast, halloumi cheese on the side

- Rooibos tea or herbal (especially liquorice) tea.

Mid-morning snacks

- 1 or 2 tablespoons of cottage cheese. Add a little chopped pineapple or a few dates, or, if you have a savoury tooth, chopped tomatoes and fresh herbs

- A small portion of cheese and grapes

- A hard-boiled egg and mayonnaise

- Discs of thickly sliced cucumber with blobs of hummus

- Oat biscuits with chicken liver paté, salmon paté, avocado, nut butter or hummus

- A few bites of cold chicken

- Cup of herbal tea.

Lunch

- Thick homemade or fresh, shop-bought soup – such as chunky vegetable and lentils, mushroom, chicken and asparagus, broccoli and stilton, pea and ham

- Jacket potato filled with tuna and sweetcorn mayonnaise, or stir-fried courgette and oatly cream

- Frittata or Spanish omelette

- Hearty salads with

  » Organic chicken and pesto
  » Beetroot, avocado, orange slices and pecan nuts
  » Free-range ham and pears with balsamic vinegar
  » Tuna, salmon or mackerel on rocket with avocado and tiny baby potatoes, with a horseradish dressing
  » Hard-boiled eggs, soft goat's cheese and asparagus
  » Hummus and olives with olive oil and pine nuts
  » Feta and fresh figs

Afternoon snack

- Fruit with a little cheese or nuts

- A few raw salted nuts or Humus or cheese on oat biscuits

- Cashew nut butter on oat biscuits

- a (low sugar) nut and seed health bar

- 2 dessertspoons of cottage cheese and 1 chopped date.

Supper

- A hearty daal and vegetable curry

- Parmigiana served with wilted spinach

- Beetroot and radish tzatziki, coriander and asparagus

- Quinoa or brown rice with roasted vegetables

- Tabbouleh – buckwheat with finely cut onions, tomatoes, mint, parsley, pine nuts olive oil and lemon juice

- Middle Eastern-style rice dishes with brown basmati rice, lamb mince or chickpeas, dried apricots, almonds, cinnamon, finely chopped onions and fresh coriander with lemon juice and olive oil dressing

- Vegetable, prawn or chicken stir-fry with rice

- Casseroles with vegetables and rice

- Grilled oily fish (trout, wild salmon) with a salad or steamed vegetables, and baby potatoes

- Good-quality free-range pork sausages with celeriac or swede mash and roasted baby carrots and beans.

- Tofu marinated in sesame seed oil, freshly grated ginger, garlic and ginger with steamed vegetables.

Healthy dessert ideas

- One or two squares of excellent-quality dark chocolate will be absolutely fine, and very nice with a cup of peppermint tea

- Mix carob or cacao powder with some Greek yoghurt or oat cream and a little xylitol

- A handful of raw mixed nuts such as pecans, almonds, brazils and hazelnuts sprinkled over Greek yoghurt with a drizzle of honey is delicious. You can add a few cardamom seeds (not pods) for an extra lovely flavour

- Poached pears or apples with cinnamon, vanilla and cloves over Greek yoghurt.

Bed Time Snack ideas

This is a tiny snack, only about 2 tablespoonsful, but can be very helpful in getting you into a deep sleep. Some people keep a little snack next to their bed because, during the night, low blood sugars can trigger the cortisol, which triggers the sympathetic nervous system, and bang, you're awake again.

Some midnight snack ideas:

- ¼ avocado pear with a little cold turkey, chicken or tofu

- 2 spoonfuls of full fat cottage cheese with a few blueberries

- 2 oat biscuits with cashew/brazil or hazel nut butter

- A little daal

- Hot milk (dairy or non-dairy) with carob powder, or whole fresh lavender flower with a little honey.

 My favourite midnight snack recipe

A very small bowl of warm porridge oats – comforting, easy to digest and provides B vitamins, magnesium, iron, selenium and zinc.

With a generous spoonful of ground almonds – contains melatonin to support your sleep, plus protein and fat to delay gastric emptying

Whole milk or oat/almond milk – the fat keeps you full for longer

And a tiny bit of honey – lifts the blood sugars just enough to help you fall asleep.

Getting up in the night to make this is not an appealing idea, but you could make it before bed and keep it in a thermos flask besides your bed to enjoy if you wake up.

The matter of salt

An aspect of normal dietary advice that does not apply to you if you have adrenal fatigue, unless you have high blood pressure, is to maintain a low salt intake. In fact, pure natural salt is essential for our health, and will support your recovery.

Often those who suffer from adrenal fatigue have salt cravings, an unquenchable thirst and frequent urination. They may not realize that they crave salt, but may be reaching for olive or crisps for the salt content. If you feel light-headed, washed out, dizzy when you stand up, possibly have muscle cramps or difficulty sleeping, then you may feel so much better if you increase your salt intake.

When I talk about salt, I only mean unrefined sea salt or Himalayan salt. Ordinary cheap table salt falls into the category

BALANCING YOUR BLOOD SUGAR

of junk food and will not be supportive to your health. Salt not only helps the aldosterone to hold fluid in the body, but it provides many essential minerals and electrolytes, and so it is important that you only use either unrefined sea or Himalayan salt. The Himalayan salt option is probably better because it isn't contaminated with the pollutants that unfortunately sea salt will be. Hopefully with our environmental consciousness, the seas will be cleaned up shortly – and not before time.

Copious urination and thirst may also suggest diabetes, so please do check with your doctor.

For those people who describe this intense and unquench-able thirst, I find that liquorice herb tea with a small pinch of unrefined sea or Himalayan salt significantly helps to hold the water in the body and the person quickly stops feeling so unsteady and dizzy. I particularly like to use a piece of concentrated liquorice juice stick dissolved in water with a pinch of unrefined sea, or Himalayan salt. Those who have high blood pressure should not take this tea, but most people with chronic fatigue or adrenal fatigue actually have low blood pressure.

Salt and insomnia

Here is interesting a nugget that may come as a surprise. Insomnia can be related to a low salt diet. Because of the weakened adrenal glands, the aldosterone struggles to hold the fluid and the blood volume drops, this triggering the sympathetic nervous system to secrete those hormones of stress – cortisol and adrenaline,[1] and of course, you can't sleep.

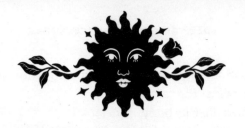

CHAPTER 4

DEEP AND RESTORATIVE SLEEP

This is the awful irony about people with adrenal fatigue: they are utterly exhausted, and yet they can't sleep.

All through the day and the early evening they feel limp and weak, but they keep soldiering on, because that is the sort of person they are. Then, a miracle occurs! The clock strikes eleven and, TING – they wake up! Suddenly there is the energy that they have lacked all through the day, and so they buzz around getting things done and often don't go to bed until around 2 or 3 a.m. Others are "wired and tired", and just cannot fall asleep, or they may fall asleep, only to wake suddenly in the night.

My experience of helping people with chronic fatigue is that the sleeping pattern can be one of the most difficult problems to crack, but below are a few tips which I hope you will find helpful.

Get to bed early enough

Many people who have become ill due to too much stress are goal-orientated or achievement-driven, and they can feel that they ought to be enjoying evening activities. Frequently people say to me: "I can't just work – I need to have a life in the evenings too."

Others feel that although they cannot be very productive during the day, when their brain wakes up at night, they want to take advantage of it. This is all completely understandable, but I also argue that it is wiser to listen to your body rather than your mind. Sometimes the mind is a very hard taskmaster, and the body just cannot keep up.

Try to be in bed by 9 p.m. with a lovely warm drink and a gentle book or music to soothe your mind. If you do choose to watch television, steer away from the rampant misery which the TV companies feed their audiences, and aim more towards gentler, uplifting programmes. Don't read thrillers before bed because, exciting as they are, they are also difficult to put down. Screens are stimulating too. There is plenty of evidence to suggest that their blue light suppresses melatonin production in the brain and thus makes sleeping more difficult.

Instead, read something gentle, kindly and even something slightly boring. A lot of people find books on meditation or other such kindly peaceful subjects to be excellent bedtime reading. Then you will find that your mind slows down before that watershed hour of 11 p.m., you have dropped your book and slipped into a restful slumber. The idea is that in time, this routine will help to re-set your internal clock back to a more sociable pattern. If you allow yourself to become a night owl, the pattern becomes very hard to break and it can become a very isolating way of life. I've known people to stay awake until 3 a.m. but only get up the next day in the afternoon, and this is a very difficult pattern to break, as well as being difficult to fit back into the world – I think that I can hear some of you saying hooray for that, but it's a lonely existence.

If you have struggled to sleep for months or years, when you do finally start to have regular, full nights' sleep, you will probably wake in the morning feeling even more tired than before. Don't worry; this is quite normal. Now that your body is finally able to let go, it is resting and recovering. After a few weeks of catching up, the tiredness will lift and you will feel so much better again.

Sometimes the most restorative sleep is from 6 to 10 a.m. This is quite a common pattern with adrenal fatigue. If you are able to, do allow yourself this time to sleep, but be very careful to make sure that you get into bed by 9 p.m., so that you do not start a new pattern of "late to bed, late to get up".

I myself have suffered from adrenal fatigue a few times, and at those times I have been very happy to get home from work, eat supper, run a bath and then get into bed with a book by 7:30 p.m.! I won't fall asleep for hours, but as I happily read my book, I am snug and quiet, and I recover. I have to recover because I have my lovely patients to heal.

Keep a snack next to your bed

As I explained in chapter 3 (Balancing your blood sugar), often people wake during the night because their blood sugar levels have dropped. This causes the cortisol to shoot up and then they are awake. You might like to keep a snack next to your bed so that you don't have to get up and rummage through the fridge, waking yourself up, but often, a snack before you fall asleep can make the difference between a full night's sleep or waking with a start at 2 a.m. Just something like almond butter on an oat cake, or the oat and almond porridge which I mentioned at the end of the last chapter, kept warm and ready for you in a thermos flask.

Keep calm but don't carry on

Some people find that they can't fall asleep because their mind is whirling with all the things they need to do tomorrow (achieving again), or worries/excitements of the day gone by. There are ways to cope with these problems, such as keeping a note book which you allows you to draw up a to-do list, so that you don't need to think about or remember the jobs. Keep the to-do list realistic.

You might even choose to prepare a weekly roster, so that you know what will be achieved, but making sure that some "me-time" has been scheduled into the week. This way, you won't have to worry that such and such won't be achieved, because you can see that it will be achieved, but in bite-sized portions. Do make sure that these goals are small and achievable and that you respect your energy boundaries.

As you recover your strength and health, you can take on more again. I cannot emphasize enough that it really matters that you rest and pace yourself. Give up worrying about achieving. Try to give up worrying. I always tell my patients who worry about their recovery programme: "Please don't worry about your herbs and your treatment programme. That is for me to be concerned about. Just rest, eat well and sleep well. And take your herbs. Try to be happy and think about the things that make your heart sing – then do those things."

Bathing therapy

We all know that warm water is very therapeutic. When you are exhausted and your muscles ache, lying in a warm bath of water takes the weight off your body for a while and allows the muscles to unravel. You can exalt your bath time with essential oils help soothe your mind and body.

Have a lovely warm bath with essential oils, then wrap yourself up in a fluffy dressing gown and toddle off softly to bed. The vaporized essential oils enter the emotional part of your brain (the limbic system) directly from your nose, quietening the central nervous system. Even if you have lost your sense of smell, your brain and body will respond.

If you don't have a bath, you can simply make a foot bath. Fill a little tub with warm water, add the same recipes as below and soak your feet in the healing waters. Keep some hot water next to you to top up if the water cools too much, and make sure that you cover your legs with a towel, which is very useful when you want to take your feet out of the water. You might even like to have a hot water bottle at your lower back or shoulders. While you are relaxing, you can enjoy a herbal tea and read a gentle book, meditate or listen to some soothing music. Take this time out just for yourself, to quieten your mind and prepare for bed. After about 30 minutes, dry off, tuck your toes into some cosy socks, and pad off to bed.

Relaxing bath oils

In a little container, combine 1 tablespoon of base oil (even kitchen olive oil is fine) with the following essential oils.

 Joyful floral blend

4 drops of rose geranium essential oil
6 drops of roman chamomile essential oil
4 drops of petitgrain essential oil
6 drops of ylang-ylang essential oil

 A steadying, grounding blend

6 drops of lavender essential oil
2 drops of vetiver essential oil
5 drops of frankincense essential oil
6 drops of cedar wood essential oil

This is a lovely blend when you have spent too much time whizzing around the mental sphere, and long to sink into forest and the deep earth.

Salt bath

An Epsom salt bath is even better. The magnesium minerals seep into tight muscles, relieving pain, pulling out toxins, and allowing the mind to let go.

Peaceful and uplifting bath salts

4 drops of lavender essential oil
4 drops of cedar essential
6 drops of frankincense essential oil
6 drops petitgrain essential oil
1 tablespoon of a base oil
2 handfuls of Epsom salts

Mix up all the oils and salts well, then toss the whole lot into your bath. Get in quickly and lie with your shoulders deeply submerged for at least 20 minutes. Keep a glass of cold water next to you, so that you can hydrate at the same time. When you emerge, wrap up warmly and enjoy a peaceful evening.

 ## A sea bath

A more unusual type of bath is a seaweed bath, which feels very like a spa experience. Mix two handfuls of Dead Sea Salts with a tablespoon of Kelp powder, and tip into your bath tub. Your bathroom will smell very richly of the sea, and you will feel a relaxing yet revitalizing effect as the mineral-rich waters soak into your skin.

Foot massage

This is a lovely routine to perform for yourself or someone else at bedtime. Castor oil has been used since ancient Egyptian times to provide a deeply restful sleep. It is a thick syrupy oil, which warms the tissues, relieves pain and tenderness in muscles, increases blood flow and reduces inflammation in the joints and nervous tissues.

1. Pour boiling water into a tiny ceramic bowl to warm it. Then throw out the water.

2. Add 2 teaspoons of castor oil, 2 drops of lavender essential oil, and 2 drops of frankincense essential oil.

3. Now, take this to your bedroom and gently massage each foot with a little of the blend, paying special attention to the parts of the foot that are asking for extra attention. You might like to look up a reflexology chart and see which part of the body that area on your foot corresponds to. Then, pull on some comfy socks and slip into bed. After about an hour, you can remove your socks and you won't spoil your sheets because the oils will have been absorbed by your feet.

Herbs which calm nerves and promote sleep

There are many herbs which can be used to calm the nerves, and these form one of the cornerstones of your recovery programme.

It can be quite beneficial to take calming herbs in the early evening before supper, so that the herbs have had a chance to quieten your mind some hours before you fall asleep. This is especially helpful if your head is still whizzing from a busy day.

Passionflower (*Passiflora incarnata*)

This is one of the most popular herbs for those who feel anxious and jittery through the day. It is a very safe herb, which leaves one feeling beautifully peaceful. It can give the feeling of slight euphoria, but I think this is simply the immense joy at feeling peaceful and calm if you have felt anxious for an extended period of time. *Passiflora* is in no way stimulating, and you can take it in small doses through the day as well as at night to help you drop off to sleep.

Valerian (*Valeriana officinalis*)

This is one of my favourite herbs to use when people feel overwhelmed with too much to do. When you can't see the wood for the trees, valerian quietens the mind and allows mental clarity. Valerian seems to create a little distance between the aggravating circumstance and yourself, which gives you a moment to draw breath before responding. I have used it many times when someone has arrived at my clinic, tight with tension. I give them 5ml, and soon they are smiling and calm.

It is an immensely peaceful herb but be aware that a very small percentage of people find that it makes them even more jittery. If you are one of those people, then you must just leave it alone, because you will always have this reaction to it.

Vervain (*Verbena officinalis*)

There is a lovely old saying which says that "Vervain is as comforting as a mother's hug." This herb can be used when one is fretful and disturbed, but not completely overwhelmed. I find it particularly helpful for menopausal women as it has a mild oestrogenic effect as well. Vervain helps you to feel more settled and comfortable in your world.

Lemon balm (*Melissa officinalis*)

Lemon balm is a very common garden plant which works best when it is freshly picked and popped into a teapot of boiling water. It calms the nerves and lifts the spirits. Just add one large sprig to a cup of boiling water. Cover with a saucer until you are ready to drink, then enjoy a light lemony infusion. Please do avoid this herb if you have an underactive thyroid, as it decreases the production of thyroid hormone in the gland.

Californian poppy (*Eschscholzia californica*)

Californian poppy is used to relax the mind and soothe nerve pain. It helps promote sleep, eases nervous agitation, and is particularly renowned for helping those who are sensitive to changes in the weather. I particularly like to use it for those who find sleep difficult because of pain.

Rose (*Rosa damascene*)

Beautiful rose – the herb of the heart. This herb reduces cortisol, and calms and soothes emotional pain. If there is heartache, emotional exhaustion and turbulence, this herb brings peace and comfort.

When using herbals, I always suggest that it would be so much safer and more effective for you to consult a professional medical herbalist. They will also not only offer the most appropriate herb for you, but almost certainly include others, such as adrenal-supporting herbs, immune tonics, and hormonal-regulating herbs, etc. Most of all, herbs are the tools of the herbalist's trade and you will judge her according to the results of her treatment, so she will only prescribe the best quality herbs. The quality of a herbal product is not always the top priority in supermarkets or the internet.

Nutritional supplements which calm nerves and promote sleep

Magnesium

About 70% of the population is deficient in magnesium. It is a very useful mineral to bring into your home treatment programme because it plays such an integral part in the whole-body system., being a cofactor for over 300 enzyme systems which regulate our body function. Magnesium is particularly helpful for the nervous system and our muscles.

Taking magnesium has been shown to significantly increase sleep time, possibly because it raises the melatonin levels in the brain.[1] It also plays a huge role in regulating muscle contractions, and is thus the first thing that I will think about using when considering how to ease restless leg syndrome, muscle spasms, tight shoulders and headaches originating from the neck.

It can also be very useful for those who suffer from constipation due to what used to be called a spastic colon. Anxiety-related irritable bowel syndrome may also respond positively to a magnesium supplement.

Foods rich in magnesium include:

- Oats

- Kelp

- Pumpkin seeds

- Almonds

- Cashew nuts

There probably isn't enough magnesium in food to top up our common deficiency, however, and I find that magnesium citrate or maleate really can help support sleep and muscle pain. However, sometimes the tablets are not well absorbed, in which case you can try liquid magnesium, which tastes awful but is very efficiently absorbed into the body.

Calcium

Calcium, especially when contained in food, has a calming and sedative effect on the body. A calcium deficiency in the body is associated with a more restless sleep. Calcium and magnesium taken 45 minutes before bedtime have a nice calming effect.

Foods rich in calcium include:

- Yoghurt

- Cheese

- Broccoli

- Tinned sardines (by eating the soft bones)

- Sesame seeds

- Tahini

Vitamin B complex

A vitamin B complex is one of my go-to supplements for those who feel debilitated from nervous exhaustion. Vitamin B is well known to nourish and support the nervous system, particularly for people who have been under tremendous stress for a long time. All this stress draws on the nervous system, which needs extra nourishment. Foods rich in B vitamins include:

- Oats

- Cashew nuts

- Brazil nuts

- Hazelnuts

- Walnuts

- Pecans

Organ meats such as liver pate on oat biscuits, fried liver and oranges on a rocket salad, egg yolks, brown rice. However, once again, I think that a good vitamin B complex supplement for a short period of time can be very helpful.

Tryptophan

This is an amino acid which is converted into serotonin in the brain, and thus enhances the brain's ability to produce melatonin, the hormone which regulates your body's natural inner clock. Thus, trytophan helps to promote a healthy sleep pattern. L-tryptophan is found in foods such as milk and turkey. Milk and dairy products such as cheese, particularly Swiss cheese, contain the highest amount of tryptophan available in a food.

 Bedtime drinks

For a calming, comforting bedtime drink, warm some dairy or cashew/almond milk, add a little honey and float a flower head of lavender in it.

For a tasty oaty bedtime drink, warm half a mug of water with half a mug of oat milk. Take 1 tablespoon of porridge oats and whizz them in a coffee grinder to a powder. Stir the oat powder into the warming milk and grate a little nutmeg into the mixture. Add half a teaspoon of vanilla extract or 1 drop of vanilla essence, and sweeten – with a little stevia or xylitol if you are avoiding sugar, honey for comfort, or, if you want to go back to the days of your childhood nursery, a little golden syrup or maybe even a tiny knob of butter.

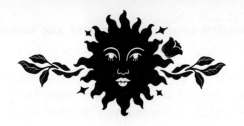

CHAPTER 5

SUPPORTING YOUR DIGESTION

In earlier chapters, I described how stress diverts the nervous system away from the parasympathetic "rest and digest" pathway towards the sympathetic "fight and flight" pathway, causing the muscles in the gut to contract into irritable bowel–type spasms, and at the same time shutting down the secretion of digestive acids and enzymes. It makes sense – when we are running away or in a fight, eating is not on our mind. Once the drama is over, a little while later, we may be famished, but in the heat of the moment, we do not think about eating.

In our modern life, when we live and eat in a constant hurry, food is gulped down instead of being thoroughly chewed and mixed with saliva. These large chunks of food hit the stomach, but without sufficient hydrochloric acid in the stomach and enzymes in the small intestine, the food cannot be digested sufficiently. It feels like a brick in the stomach, and in that warm, moist environment it ferments, producing lots of gas so that the person feels bloated and uncomfortable. The fermenting bacteria create toxins as a by-product, which inflame the gut lining, leading to large holes in the gut lining known as "gut permeability". These gaps in the intestinal lining allow undigested food particles to leak into the bloodstream. The immune cells circulating in the blood are familiar with small completely digested food molecules such as amino acids, but large, partially digested proteins such as polypeptides are not recognized, and are seen as invaders by the immune system, and thus the cells attack these molecules, and in doing so, set up food intolerances.

This undesirable situation can be further compounded by a high-sugar diet. When people are very tired, they naturally want to eat sugar to give them energy. A little bit of sugar is fine, but when a treat becomes a daily habit, problems quickly develop. Yeasts live in small populations within our gut; however, when too much sugar is added to the dark, moist environment, the yeast population absolutely explodes. (Think how quickly mushrooms can pop up on a lawn overnight.) In a favourable environment, these yeasts quickly grow root-like mycelia, which penetrate the gut wall, causing further gut permeability (leaky gut). Now the partially digested food particles and the yeast cells slip through the gaps in the gut wall into the bloodstream. The patrolling immune system in the blood doesn't recognize the yeasts, nor the large undigested food particles, and immediately attacks them, because that is its job. In this way the immune system becomes sensitized to these foods and systemic candidiasis develops.

As a result of always having to attack these food particles and yeasts, the immune system becomes weary, and with stress, high levels of cortisol are also damping down the immune response. The simultaneously exhausted and suppressed immune system starts to confuse the body's own tissues with the large particles of food proteins which should not be floating about in the bloodstream, and so it begins to attack the body tissues as well – often resulting in joint pains. The yeast cells then progress into the joints, depositing toxins, making the joint pain worse. It progresses into the brain, causing brain fog, and into the sinuses, causing sinus congestion. The person becomes more and more tired, headachy, and frequently resorts to sugar and caffeine to keep going. The end result can be autoimmune conditions.

The damage caused by stress is extremely harmful to the body, but it is repairable. Once again, I strongly advise you to see a naturopathic practitioner. In the meantime, there is a great deal that you can do to heal your own body.

Rest and digest

We were not designed to eat on the hoof. When do you ever see a San Bushman running while eating his steak? Never! He has the good sense to sit down with his family under the stars and tell wonderful stories about the animals he encounters, while eating his food at a leisurely pace. In doing so, he allows the correct pathway of his nervous system to prepare his gut to digest his food.

We don't have the luxury of time in our money-rich, time-poor lives, but do try your very best to eat in a civilized manner. Not long ago we all sat down at a regular time, to eat as a family at the dining room table. We did not take phone calls or watch television, and arguments during mealtimes were frowned upon. There was a lot of wisdom in that.

Many of us don't have dining rooms anymore, but we can prepare our own meals. The smells of cooking enthuses our digestive systems to receive the food, and the slowness of cooking is in itself a quiet time. Then sitting with your family or friends – with gentle music, candles if you wish, and convivial conversation is one of life's pleasantries.

Relax the gut

Many people don't outwardly show their stress or anxiety, but feel it acutely in their guts. There are some wonderful herbs which really help to relax these sometimes crippling spasms. It is easy to find German chamomile, fennel, peppermint or spearmint and ginger teas in the supermarket, and these are absolutely fabulous at relaxing those tight, cramping stomach muscles, and will also encourage the secretions of digestive enzymes. Herbs like melissa and catnip relax the mind and the gut, and can be grown in your garden or even in a pot on a windowsill.

 Relaxing tummy tea

Drop 1 bag of chamomile tea, 1 bag of peppermint tea and 1 bag of fennel tea into a mug. Inhale the fragrant steam while the hot water cools, then drink the tea.

 Digestive tea

Pop 1 bag of chamomile tea, 2 sprigs of fresh mint, ½ tsp of fennel or caraway seeds, 5 slices of fresh ginger root and 1 slice of lemon into a tea pot of boiling water and allow to brew for 10 minutes. Strain and sip gently whilst relaxing. Perhaps you could make a ritual of it with deeply relaxing music, or lying on your bed with a magazine and soft lighting. Make a special moment of your herb tea.

Encourage digestive enzymes

Even in the 1900s, it was normal practice that when you sat down to a meal at a hotel, you were placed at a table with a starched white table cloth and a small glass of pineapple juice or half a grapefruit before you began your meal. This was not just a nicety, but good for your digestion, as the fruit juices trigger the release of digestive enzymes.

People with chronic fatigue often are not able to produce enough hydrochloric acid (stomach acid). Hydrochloric acid helps to break down foods into their smaller absorbable molecules, and also assists in the absorption of nutrients and kills unwanted bacteria in the digestive tract. We can feel bloated, gassy or even have heartburn.

Some people are so debilitated that their bodies do not even have the energy to digest their food, or their body seems to have "forgotten" how to secrete the right enzymes. I have seen this in very ill people where their digestive system shuts down, and the food seems to run right through them. For those people, small meals are the only ones that the body can manage, and even then, supplementary digestive enzymes are going be a necessity for a while, until the body has been restored to health.

In these cases, the body has to be re-trained to secrete the enzymes using herbs. It has to be nourished with small, highly nutritious meals, and those nutrients have to be made available to the body via digestive enzyme capsules until it is able to take over that function again.

As a medical herbalist, I would prescribe digestive enzymes for a while, to help my patients digest their food, but I would also teach them how to eat, to support this all-important digestive process. Here are some of my top tips to get those digestive juices flowing again:

- Squeeze half a lemon into a small glass of water and sip half an hour before a meal to encourage the liver to secrete bile, which digests fats.

- Add bitter foods such as rocket, radishes or chicory salad to your salads, which will encourage the digestive tract to secrete enzymes., so try adding some to your salad mix.

- Incorporate fragrant herbs such as thyme, oregano and sage act through the olfactory system, alerting the brain that there is something delicious to eat, and the brain will send a message to the stomach to prepare for this food. Fragrant herbs can be added to your casseroles, roasts and salads, snipped over potatoes, and into rice and quinoa dishes.

- Fresh fruits contains enzymes which break down foods, but these enzymes are destroyed with heat, so you need to eat the fruit raw. A great way to help digest your food is to have a portion of fruits, with a dollop of live plain yoghurt after a main meal.

Foods naturally rich in digestive enzymes

- **Kiwi fruit** contains actinidin, which digests proteins

- **Avocado** contains lipase, which digests fat

- **Banana** contains amylase and maltase, which help to digest carbohydrates

- **Mango** contains amylase, which breaks down starches into sugars

- **Papaya** contains papain, which digests proteins

- **Pineapple** contains bromelain, which breaks down proteins

- **Ginger** contains zingibain, which aids protein digestion and encourages the secretion of other digestive enzymes.

If you feel that you struggle to digest your food, make sure it is well cooked. Raw vegetables and salads are rich in cellulose, which is indigestible, but the cooking process breaks it down, making the nutrients available to your cells. When one is very ill, you need warm food in an easily digestible state, so I suggest soft proteins like fish or eggs, and soft vegetables which have been steamed. Hearty soups made with bone broth are absolute winners when it comes to bringing nutrition to an exhausted body.

Encourage regular bowel movements

Stress can cause the muscles in the colon to seize up with anxiety. In the old days, this used to be called spastic colon, and the result is that the natural peristalsis does not occur. If the large bowel does not contract and empty the faecal matter regularly, the toxins in the faeces start to leach back through the colon wall into the bloodstream, inflaming the intestinal lining and leading to toxins being deposited in the cells. The liver becomes clogged up, leading to poor detoxification of the blood, which can cause headaches, lethargy, bad breath and skin problems.

We have already discussed how the bowel needs to be relaxed, but it also needs to be encouraged to empty. If there is enough roughage and fluid in the contents of the faeces, these will swell slightly, causing the walls of the large intestine to be gently dilated. This gentle stretch stimulates the muscles of the bowel to contract in a coordinated manner – in other words, it will stimulate a bowel movement.

Whole grains such as brown rice, porridge oats, fresh vegetables and legumes will provide ample healthy fibre in your diet, but if that is not enough, there is another trick. One of the simplest and healthiest ways of encouraging a bowel movement is to include flaxseeds or chia seeds in your diet. When these seeds are introduced to the gut, they absorb the fluid in the digestive tract, and also capture any toxins which have been eliminated by the bile from the liver. Then this lovely slimy roughage swells in the bowel, encouraging a full and comfortable bowel movement, leaving you feeling cleansed and light in your body.

Flaxseed yoghurt

Add 1–2 dessertspoons of flaxseeds to a cup of
live plain yoghurt. You may add some prunes, fruit
or even carob powder if you wish. Then it is very
important that you immediately follow with a large
glass of warm water (or one of the herbal teas
described above). Do this every day in between
meals so as not to bind your nutrients.

 ## Chia mint water

This is refreshing and cooling on hot summer days.
    Make a cup of mint tea allow to cool, then
remove the mint, but retain the water.
    Mix 1 dessertspoon of chia seeds into the minty
water, and add a squeeze of lemon. Stir vigorously.
    Soon the seeds will begin to swell and within
an hour you will have a nice, minty, frogspawn-
like drink. Nasty as this sounds, it is actually very
cooling and soothing to drink – and your intestines
will love it.

Support the liver

Located just under the ribcage on the right side of the
abdomen, the liver is one of the largest organs in the human
body. It performs hundreds of tasks every minute of the
day – more than any other organ, including the brain! It is
constantly filtering, detoxifying, synthesizing, and processing
a wide variety of substances.

The liver also has to deal with emotions, believe it or not.
Traditional Chinese medicine states that anger causes the
liver to "stagnate" in its function of circulating the *qi* (the
vital energy of life). It is not hard to translate that into: "The

frustration and stress of our everyday lives clogs up our flow of energy."

Without a healthy, well-functioning liver, it is easy to become overly toxic, which can lead to a general feeling of lethargy, sickness and depression. In addition to its endless detoxification work, the liver is an organ that provides energy to our bodies. It does so by regulating carbohydrate and protein metabolism, hormonal activity, fat burning and blood sugar control. It is also closely linked to your digestion and secretes bile into your small intestine. The bile secreted by your liver emulsifies the fats that you eat so that they can be absorbed.

Some of my patients complain of a feeling of "not being able to digest fat". Others tell me that they feel poisoned. Food choices, environmental toxins, unfriendly bacteria and yeasts all contribute towards a congested and fatigued liver, but there are some herbs and foods that can support the gallbladder and liver to be able to do their jobs again.

- Have a glass of hot water with a slice of lemon and fresh ginger first thing in the morning. This will give the liver a nice little morning flush and helps encourage digestive enzymes.

- Organic vegetables have become much more affordable these days, so it is possible to reduce your intake of the remnants of pesticide toxins.

- If you can manage, do try to eat organic or at least free-range meat and eggs. Less, high quality meat is healthy for everyone and the planet.

- Fibre-rich foods help to cleanse the bowel, decongest the colon and thus relieve the liver of a toxic load.

- Drastically reduce (or, ideally, completely stop) indulging in alcohol, coffee, soft drinks and refined sugar of any kind.

- Drink plenty of water or herbal teas to flush the cells, blood and lymph of toxins, thereby relieving the liver of a toxic burden.

Foods to naturally support your liver

- **Garlic** has the ability to activate the liver enzymes that help your body flush out toxins. It also contains high amounts of allicin and selenium, two natural compounds that aid in liver cleansing, and at the same time it is a fabulous anti-fungal, anti-bacterial and anti-viral vegetable.

- **Grapefruit** is high in both vitamin C and antioxidants, and increases the natural cleansing processes of the liver. A small glass of freshly squeezed grapefruit juice will help boost production of liver detoxification enzymes that help flush toxins.

- **Beetroot** and **carrots** are both extremely high in plant flavonoids and beta-carotene, and . Eating both beetroot and carrots can help stimulate and improve overall liver function.

- **Green tea** – this liver-loving beverage is bursting with plant antioxidants known as catechins, a constituent known to assist the liver's overall functions.

- **Leafy green vegetables** are our most powerful allies in cleansing the liver, and can be eaten raw, cooked or juiced. Extremely high in plant chlorophylls, leafy greens literally suck up environmental toxins from the bloodstream. With their distinct ability to neutralize heavy metals, chemicals and pesticides, these cleansing foods offer a powerful protective mechanism for the liver.

- **Avocados** are a nutrient-dense superfood which help the body produce glutathione, necessary for the liver to cleanse harmful toxins.

- **Apples** are high in pectin, which helps the body to cleanse and release toxins from the digestive tract. This, in turn, makes it easier for the liver to handle the toxic load in the body.

- **Walnuts** are high in glutathione and omega-3 fatty acids, which support normal liver cleansing actions. Make sure you chew the nuts well (until they are liquefied) before swallowing.

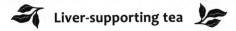 **Liver-supporting tea**

Put 3 slices of fresh ginger root (or ¼ tsp of dried ginger powder), 3 slices of fresh turmeric root (or ¼ tsp of dried turmeric powder), ½ tsp of dried dandelion root and 1 sprig of fresh rosemary in a teapot and leave to steep for 30 minutes before straining. Drink twice a day.

Restore your microbiome

Let's talk about your bugs. Our body is made up of over 50 trillion cells, and within our guts live 100 trillion microbes, of which around 90% are bacteria, and the rest are fungi and archaea. There are approximately another 50 trillion living in your nose, on your skin, in the vagina, ears, etc. It turns out, we are less of a single organism and more of an environmental system. While we used to think of these entities as separate from ourselves, just hanging out in our gut, but we now know that this is not the case at all.

Microbes form a whole body system in their own right, and we cannot live without each other, so we must look after them. The microbes in our gut have an extremely influential role in our immunity – both training our body to attack invaders and damping down inappropriate inflammation. They play an essential part in resisting invading bacteria and viruses, maintaining the health of our gut barrier and metabolizing nutrients. Cross-talking between our gut and our nervous system even affects our mood. The gut bacteria produce about 95% of our serotonin, so if the microbiome is disrupted, it could result in anxiety or depression.

We don't know how many strains of bacteria, fungi and archaea live within our gut, but there are probably thousands of strains, and the population changes daily according to our diet. With their direct influence on our health, that means that we can influence our immunity and wellbeing with the food that we eat.

When the microbial population becomes disrupted by too many unfriendly bacteria, or the yeast population explodes, we say that there is dysbiosis, which is an umbrella term for a collection of microbial-disrupted-associated illnesses such as SIBO (Small Intestinal Bacterial Overgrowth), candidiasis, irritable bowel syndrome, inflammatory bowel disease, and others such as rheumatoid arthritis. A very recent study has shown a "microbial signature" for people with CFS/ME, demonstrating that fatigue and gut bacteria can have a direct relationship.[1]

Let's have a look at some of the symptoms associated with some dysbiotic conditions:

Yeast overgrowth

- Gas, flatulence and stomach bloating

- Itchy scalp

- Athlete's foot and other fungal infections

- Itchy vagina, penis and/or anus

- Discharge from the vagina or the penis

- Brain fog

- Aching joints

- Hormonal imbalance.

SIBO (small intestinal bacterial overgrowth)

- Abdominal bloating, pain and distention

- Nausea

- Diarrhoea

- Fatigue and weakness

- Burping

- Joint pain

- Skin rashes

- Hormonal imbalances.

Dysbiosis in the colon

- Bloating

- Flatulence

- Bad breath

- Rashes

- Brain fog, lethargy and fatigue

- Diarrhoea and/or constipation

- Abdominal cramping

- Mucous and/or blood in the stool

- Depression and/or anxiety.

If you recognize these symptoms, at the very least you should avoid all sugary foods, which feed the unfriendly bugs. While starving the yeasts and unfriendly bacteria, you can vastly improve your diet by including plenty of vegetables and protein such as oily fish, legumes, organic eggs and nuts.

Next, you need to kill the unfriendly invaders. Herbalists have strong herbs to do this job, but your kitchen cupboard has excellent options too.

Raw garlic is a really powerful anti-microbial. It can make you feel a bit queasy, so I recommend that you mash it avocado and eat this on rye toast, or rub it onto rye toast, then add slices of raw tomato and drizzle olive oil on top for a delicious breakfast. You might like it crushed into lemon juice and olive oil as a salad dressing, or mix it into mashed potato.

Note: don't eat raw garlic for longer than about four days without changing to something else, because it is a bit harsh on the gut lining, and if you ever feel that it burns your stomach, stop eating it immediately.

Another good option is cinnamon, which is anti-fungal and anti-bacterial. Simply add half a teaspoon of cinnamon powder to a cup of boiling water and sip – on an empty stomach, this time.

Probiotics and prebiotics

Probiotics are widely available on the market, and it is very important that you buy yours from a reputable company. I buy mine from a laboratory which only makes probiotics (rather than a wide range of vitamin and mineral supplements), as their entire focus and reputation rests on the quality of their bacteria.

Although friendly bacteria are found in live or bio yoghurts, their numbers are small. They still do have a beneficial effect on the gut microbial population, but these products do not carry enough bacteria to have the therapeutic impact that probiotic capsules do. The probiotic industry is becoming increasingly sophisticated with specific bacterial strains to support the microbiome of the bladder, moderate histamine production or support the mood. To achieve these results you need high quality professional probiotics.

However, as a day to day treat, live plain yoghurt with fresh or stewed fruit is an excellent option to help maintain a healthy microbiome. The flavoured yoghurts may be very tasty, but have far too much sugar in them, and those little probiotic drinks also tend to be very high in sugar.

Other probiotic foods include kefir, sauerkraut and kimchi, kombucha and a soy product called natto.

Probiotic bacteria are little animals, and so they need to be fed. The food they eat is called prebiotics. Foods rich in prebiotics include slippery elm, onions, asparagus, Jerusalem artichokes, apples, legumes and wholegrains.

Saccharomyces boulardii is a yeast probiotic which helps to kill and flush out other unfriendly bacteria and yeasts by preventing them from adhering to the gut wall. Even though it is a yeast, it is a friendly yeast, and works very well with the probiotic bacteria.

Taking a probiotic supplement, along with avoiding sugar and eating healthy foods, and drinking cinnamon tea is an effective and a safe way to help redress the balance of your gut microbiome. The more varied the diet, the more strains of healthy bacteria you introduce to your gut, means that you will crowd out the unfriendly bacteria and yeast which cause the bloating, flatulence, bowel toxins and the symptoms associated with those. The friendly bacteria can then start to repair the gut wall and your immune system, rebuilding your health from a strong foundation.

 Stewed apples with yogurt

2 apples
½ tsp of cinnamon
2 cloves
A small knob of organic butter
Just a little water

Core the apples, but leave the skin on, and chop into pieces. Drop into a small saucepan. Sprinkle the cinnamon, add the cloves. Put a little water in the saucepan, and add the butter. Put the lid on and turn the heat onto low. Keep checking the water, so that the apples don't burn. In about 10 minutes the shapes of apple pieces will be softened but not completely collapsed. Take the pan off the heat, and put the stewed apples into a glass or ceramic bowl, into the fridge.

Enjoy your stewed apples with live plain yoghurt or kefir for a tummy-loving treat.

Heal the leaky gut

Food intolerances, long-term stress, yeast overgrowth, SIBO, high alcohol intake and long-term overuse of nonsteroid anti-inflammatories can inflame the gut lining and cause it to become perforated with holes, thus becoming "leaky". As a result, undigested food particles escape into the bloodstream, setting up immune responses which can cause significant health problems, like recurrent headaches (neuro-inflammation), brain fog, fatigue, joint pains and autoimmune conditions. It has now been recognized that chronic fatigue syndrome has a strong association with gut permeability and dysbiosis.[23]

If a stool test shows dysbiosis (too much of the wrong bacteria or yeast overgrowth), you can safely assume that you have a leaky gut – or if not, then an inflamed gut which is on its way to becoming permeable. Also, if you have developed food intolerances, then you will have a leaky gut.

This is where herbal medicines and nutritional supplements can help tremendously; however, there are foods and gentle herbs which you can use at home to heal the leaky gut:

- **Chamomile, calendula flowers, turmeric, marshmallow root** and **liquorice root** are all herbs that have been traditionally used to heal inflamed and leaky guts. I find that teas are the most gentle and helpful way to treat the gut, as they wash over the inflamed tissues without the aggressiveness of the alcohol found in tinctures. You should be able to buy these herbs easily from a health shop or herbal apothecary to make into a healing tea. (Do be aware, however, that liquorice can raise the blood pressure and loosen the bowels.)

- *Aloe vera* or the African *Aloe ferox* are both excellent for healing an inflamed and painful gut. Both provide the gut with healing compounds in food-state form which makes them easily acceptable and digestible to the gut, while at the same time they are soothing and anti-inflammatory to the intestinal lining. Aloe also provides prebiotics, supporting the probiotic population, as well as providing soft cellulose, which encourages regular and cleansing bowel movements.

- **Cabbage water** has long been used to heal gastric ulcers, and we seem to like science to remind us of the wisdom of those old ladies. Nowadays we can buy posh vitamin U supplements, but in the olden days, the wives would drink the water in which cabbage had been boiled to heal ulcers and inflammations of the gut as it is rich in vitamin U.

- **Butter** contains butyric acid, which provides your intestinal cells with 70% of their energy, and exerts a significant anti-inflammatory and healing effect on an inflamed intestinal lining.[4] Choose organic, grass-fed butter at the very least, but if you can, try to buy butter which comes from "calf-at-foot cows". These cows keep their calves with them until they are naturally weaned, and share their milk with the dairy. You can taste the contentment in the butter, and in doing so, you are not eating the butter of distressed cows who have had their babies stolen from them at birth.

- **Bone broth** is highly nutritious and rich in collagen, which provides the building blocks to heal a leaky gut.

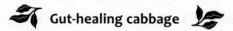 **Gut-healing cabbage**

Slice a cabbage finely and simmer in a little bone broth (or steam with water if you prefer) until just soft. Add a nice blob of butter, and a pinch of Himalayan salt, and enjoy.

- **Carob powder** is derived from large brown sweet pods of a Mediterranean tree. These pods have been used as a food since biblical times, and are still enjoyed today. Carob contains generous amounts of calcium, copper and B vitamins, and. Therapeutically, it has an effect on the gut, with both anti-diarrhoea and anti-constipation actions, as well as being anti-bacterial.[5] Carob powder is also very soothing, being anti-inflammatory, and used to heal gastric ulcers, thus absolutely fabulous to heal an inflamed, cramping leaky gut.

I love to use Carob powder for those people who are either are feeling very weak and need a nourishing drink which is easy to digest, or for those with inflamed digestive systems running from diarrhoea to constipation. It also makes a very soothing bedtime drink.

Marshmallow and carob drink

1 tsp of marshmallow root powder
1 heaped tsp of carob powder

Warm half a cup of oat/almond milk with the same amount of water in a saucepan. Whisk in and bring to a simmer. Soon the liquid will thicken into a sweet, soup-like comforting drink, which I am sure you and your intestines will absolutely love.

Take a food intolerance test

Although this is slightly diverting from our subject of stress, it really makes a great deal of sense that if you have developed a leaky gut as a result of your stressful lifestyle, then you will have developed food intolerances which will only add to your ills.

These intolerances are caused by your immune system setting up a negative reaction to certain foods which slipped through the leaky gut barrier into the bloodstream. Consequently, each time you eat these foods, the immune system goes on the attack, which is not only exhausting, but also, the immune system eventually becomes confused and starts to attack its own tissues. We think it does this because our own tissues may look similar to these large undigested food molecules, and deeper problems like autoimmune conditions can develop as a result.

If you take a test and discover that you do have food intolerances, then you need to avoid these foods for at least four to six months. During this time, it is very important that you set up a food rotation system so that you are not eating too much of another food product, thus potentially setting up a new intolerance.

These tests cost a fair amount, but are well worth it in my opinion, because you really cannot possibly guess which foods you may have become intolerant to. You might discover that you are fine with trout, but intolerant to salmon; to hazelnuts but not almonds; to cheese made from cow's milk but not goat's milk. It is well worth spending the money and even if your test results show that you have no intolerances, because that is still an answer.

Gut permeability, food intolerances and dysbiosis are some of the most important root causes of illness which appears to be of an unknown cause. A sense of calmness and healing the gut integrity are often absolutely central to the recovery process.

Healing the gut can be complicated and requires expert attention from a medical herbalist, nutritionist or dietician. However, the ideas and recipes above will go a long way towards helping to put you on the road to recovery.

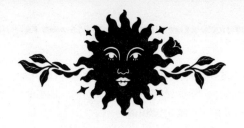

CHAPTER 6

FOODS WHICH CAUSE FATIGUE

Sometimes, it is our foods which can make us fatigued, and worse still, our favourite food can have the highest impact. Food intolerances are common, but I believe that they are usually triggered in persons who are already not very well. Whilst is well known that wheat, cow's milk and eggs may cause food intolerances (also known as food sensitivities), in fact any food can be a candidate. The difficulty in recognizing that you have food intolerances lies in the fact that the symptoms can be rather subtle. Unlike a food allergy, which is a dramatic and clear event, with food intolerance, over time you slowly develop a vague and growing sense of unwellness.

Symptoms of food intolerance

- Fatigue

- Mental fatigue and brain fog

- Bloating and abdominal cramping

- Flatulence

- Headaches

- Joint pains

- Skin rashes or itching

- Asthma or sinus congestion

- Diarrhoea

Food intolerances are caused by gut permeability, also known as "leaky gut". Sometimes foods themselves inflame the lining of the digestive system so that it becomes more permeable. An over-abundance of unfriendly bacteria, yeast over-growth such as *Candida albicans*, or other gut parasites inflame the gut and can even punch holes in the intestinal lining, thereby increasing the permeability of the gut wall.

Now, undigested food molecules are able to slip through that leaky intestinal wall into the bloodstream where they meet the circulating white blood cells. Our immune system is familiar with completely digested food particles, but the large, partially digested food molecules are marked as foreign. As such, our immune cells behave exactly as they ought to by attacking the "invader". In this way, a food intolerance is initiated. Those food molecules are remembered as invaders, and so every time you eat that particular food, the immune system will be stimulated to attack. The more you unknowingly eat that food, the more the immune system is both stimulated and exhausted by its ongoing struggle, and then something even worse can happen.

It is thought that some of the proteins in our body, for instance, those of the joint membranes, look very similar to the proteins of the undigested food molecules, which confuses the immune cells. The immune system then starts to attack its own tissues, and in doing so, initiates an autoimmune disease like rheumatoid arthritis. This mechanism, known as molecular mimicry, presents a strong theory for how autoimmune diseases develop.

There are a few ways to check for food intolerances, and my two favourites involve either a food elimination diet or a laboratory food intolerance blood test. Food intolerance tests are quite pricy but they do provide you with a swift and easy answer.

Another option is the food elimination diet. These days, food elimination diets allow plenty of vegetables and some grains, but 25 years ago, when I was taught, the patient was only allowed these 10 foods below, and nothing else.

- Lamb

- Fresh Coconut

- Pear

- Rice

- Quinoa

- Green beans

- Broccoli and cabbage

- Carrots

- Sweet potato

- Seasonings of fresh herbs and sea salt

- Olive oil

This is indeed a very strict diet to follow for a month, but naturally the more foods that you include in your elimination diet, the less chance you have of catching those foods which are the cause of your problems. Some people argue that only protein foods can cause intolerance, but my own food intolerance laboratory tests have shown pineapple, spinach and beetroot, amongst others.

When you live for a month on a strict food elimination diet, you are giving your digestive and immune system a break. It is like a gentle fast, and people often do find great relief from their symptoms, as they begin to feel healthy again.

After a month, you can start to reintroduce foods back into your diet. Every three days, you include one new food: for example, peas. That means, for three days you eat all the above foods, plus some peas. Then if you continue to feel well, you may keep peas in your diet, and you introduce another food such as Swiss chard, chicken or almonds, for instance. If you find that within the three days of introducing the new food, some of your symptoms reappear, then you know that your body is intolerant to that food item, and you should avoid it again for a while. You can try to reintroduce it again at a later date.

Whilst you are giving your digestive system a break, it is a great opportunity to introduce herbs which heal the lining of the gut. Herbal teas such as chamomile and calendula are really helpful at repairing a threadbare intestinal wall. Foods such as bone broth also provide wonderful building blocks for the intestine to use in the restoring of a healthy, strong intestinal wall.

Histamine intolerance and mast cell activation syndrome (MCAS)

There is another type of food sensitivity which is more of an allergic type, called histamine intolerance. It produces very debilitating symptoms, and dramatically impacts on one's day-to-day life.

We all have histamine in our bodies, held by cells in our bloodstream called mast cells. A commonly used metaphor for histamine intolerance is that of a bucket containing histamine. In some people, the metaphorical bucket is nearly

FOODS WHICH CAUSE FATIGUE

over-flowing with histamine. Then, if excess histamine is released because you have eaten a histamine-triggering food, have too much of the wrong type of bacteria in your small intestine, or become emotionally upset, then histamine release is initiated and the bucket overflows. The symptoms will flare because there is more histamine in the body than it is able to break down.

Symptoms of histamine intolerance

- Ongoing fatigue

- Red itchy skin

- Watery eyes and a runny nose

- Sneezing, wheezing

- Rapid heart-beat

- Low blood pressure and passing out

- Nausea

- Diarrhoea and tummy cramps

- Headaches

- Brain fog

- Depression, irritability or anxiety

Naturally, living with the above symptoms is like having a daily battle waging inside your body and it is absolutely exhausting! It is not only histamine which cause these huge inflammatory reactions. The mast cells, which are part of the white blood cell community, are like little sacs which contain a range of mediators besides histamine, called cytokines, leukotrienes and prostaglandins, and many others too.

When mast cells come into contact with an allergen such as pollen, they immediately break down (degranulate) and release their contents of inflammatory mediators, which cause our tissues to swell and flush so that our nose runs, and eyes water so that we wash the offending substance away. Thus, these mediators protect us from injury, but in the case of histamine intolerance or MCAS, the mast cells are over-sensitive, and are easily triggered to release the inflammatory molecules, thus you feel inflamed and irritated most of the time.

How do you know if you have histamine intolerance or MCAS? If you have histamine intolerance, you will respond to anti-histamine medicines, but if you have MCAS, then you won't find those medicines effective because your cells are releasing other inflammatory molecules as well.

Why people develop these conditions is not entirely clear, but possibly a genetic predisposition, coupled with other factors such as gut dysbiosis (too many unfriendly flora and fauna in your digestive tract), toxic environmental moulds, heavy metal poisoning, stress and emotional upset, or infections such as Lyme's disease, tip the balance into an inflammatory state. In short, it seems that people can be predisposed genetically, but it takes an insult to the homeostatic balance which can release a whole cascade of inflammatory molecules

This chapter only provides an introduction to a very complicated condition, which needs to be investigated more deeply, and certainly treated by a professional. Having said that, if you believe that you are histamine intolerant, you can significantly start to reduce the symptoms by following a low-histamine diet.

Foods to avoid on a low-histamine diet	Foods you may eat on a low-histamine diet
Fermented dairy: mature cheeses, yoghurt, kefir, raw milk, sour cream, buttermilk	Pasteurized A2 cow's milk, goat or sheep milk
	Non-fermented cheese such as ricotta, cottage cheese, mascarpone, paneer, mozzarella, fresh butter, cream, ghee. Home-made ice cream without artificial additives or ingredients from the high histamine list
Cured meats, bacon, cold meats, salami, sausages, leftover or aged meats, pork	Fresh meat such as chicken (no skin), beef, lamb, goat, turkey
Fish products: canned fish, smoked salmon, leftover, smoked, or salted fish, shell fish	Freshly caught fish (that day) or frozen at sea
Vegetables: green beans and peas, spinach, potato, mushrooms, aubergine, legumes, especially soy. Corn. Over-ripe fruit or vegetables, leftover food	Vegetables such as artichokes, asparagus, bell peppers, cauliflower, Swiss chard or beets, broccoli, pak choi, cabbage or brussel sprouts, fennel bulb, parsnips, carrots, garlic, cauliflower, leeks, onions, shallots, squash, turnip, courgettes, sweet potato
Fruits: grapes, dates, stone fruits such as apricots, nectarines, peaches, prunes or plums, pineapple, dried fruit, banana, papaya, strawberries, kiwi	Fruit: such as apple, pear, mango, lychees, passion fruit, rhubarb, melon, fresh fig, watermelon, fresh coconut, blueberries.
	Freshly pressed fruit juice
Salads: avocado, tomatoes, spinach	Salads: lettuce, onions, watercress, cucumber, celery, radishes, apples, raw carrots, mint
Nuts – peanuts, walnuts, pecans	Coconut and coconut milk, almonds, Brazil nuts, chia, hazelnuts, macadamia, pine-nuts
Raw egg white	Eggs (be careful, as eggs are often allergic triggers)

Yeast products such as bread, alcohol	Baked products leavened by baking powder such as soda bread, scones, muffins, biscuits, cereals without artificial additives or ingredients from the above list, rice cakes
Fermented vegetables: kimchi, sauerkraut, pickles, kombucha, vinegars, miso, natto	Rice, rice noodles, potatoes, spelt noodles, buckwheat, quinoa, amaranth, millet
Spices: star anise, cloves, curry powder or curry leaves, cinnamon, nutmeg, cayenne pepper, liquorice	Fresh herbs
Condiments: ketchup and other condiments such as tabasco sauce or mustard, soy sauce, tamari, coconut aminos, fish sauce, liquid aminos, stock cubes, gravy	
Black tea, green tea, white tea, rooibos tea	Coffee, herbal teas, natural fruit teas
Unpasteurized honey	Carob, Stevia or xylitol
Margarine, sunflower seed oil	Olive oil, coconut oil
Canned foods, food containing additives, preservatives or dyes	
Alcohol: wine, beer, champagne, cider	White spirits such as gin or vodka

Rules of thumb for a low-histamine diet

- Try as much as you can to buy organic and very fresh food, which you prepare yourself.
- Buy little and often and use the foods when very fresh.
- Keep food in the fridge or freezer.
- Try not to have left overs, and if you do, then freeze.
- Avoid canned foods, processed or ready meals.
- Avoid ripened and fermented foods.

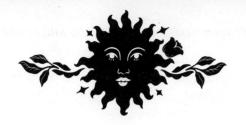

CHAPTER 7

RESTORE YOUR ADRENAL GLANDS

Restoring the adrenal glands to optimum health is one of the hubs around which we focus to bring you back to optimal health and vitality after too much stress. This is not something that happens quickly, and it is realistic to expect recovery to take anywhere from six to nine months at least – sometimes a lot longer if the person is severely debilitated.

Before I prescribe herbs for the adrenal glands, it can be helpful to run an adrenal stress test. This test can be performed in your own home and requires four samples of saliva over a typical day. The laboratory charts two adrenal hormone levels to show you if your adrenal output is above or below average range.

In healthy people, cortisol shows a sharp rise in the morning within half an hour of waking, and this is to promote wakeful alertness. After that, cortisol levels slowly drift down to a low level, so that in the evening you are ready for sleep. In some people, we see elevated cortisol levels right through the day, and this suggests a continuous stress response. Very often, people are so used to feeling stressed that they are not even aware of it, and these results can come as quite a shock.

In time, if you live under constant stress, the adrenal glands become debilitated, and the cortisol levels fall and remain below the average. I have frequently seen adrenal charts where the cortisol barely manages much of a morning peak at all, demonstrating quite clearly that the adrenal glands are deeply fatigued, and struggling to produce the cortisol necessary for a healthy lifestyle.

Having the adrenal test results can be validating. If you have felt unwell or just plain run down, constantly tired and a bit low, but with no specific symptoms to tell your doctor about, these results can give you something to work with. When you have been told for months or years that there is nothing wrong with you, it is strangely reassuring to have results in black and white. At least you have a starting point from which to begin your recovery programme. More than that, it can be a bit of a wake-up call, and can make you realize that your lifestyle is having a rather serious impact on your health and that things need to change. The test results urge you to seriously start taking care of yourself, and it is quite helpful for partners to see these results too. I am afraid that there is little point in showing your doctor these adrenal test results because currently they do not get involved with adrenal health unless you have a cancer, Cushings or Addison's disease, although quite likely, dare I say – most doctors are probably adrenally fatigued themselves.

A five-pronged approach to adrenal recovery

1. Keep your blood sugar levels even, and eat highly nourishing foods.

2. Sleep long enough and deeply enough.

3. Develop self-nurturing rituals and allow yourself the time to rest and reflect on your life, or to smell the roses, listen to the birds, or watch the clouds sail past.

4. Use herbal medicines which act as tonics and restoratives for the adrenal glands.

5. Provide the adrenal glands with the correct nutrition, which acts as building blocks, allowing recovery.

Every person who suffers from adrenal fatigue or chronic fatigue will have a slightly different case history, and as you have probably heard many times before, there is no one-size-fits-all programme for recovery. It is especially important to bear in mind that herbs and supplements can be dangerous if given in the wrong context, combined with other medication, or in incorrect doses. Thus, I urge you to consult a qualified and experienced medical herbalist or nutritional therapist/dietician before taking any natural medications so that you have someone with an in-depth knowledge of the natural medicines, and physiology and pathology, guiding you through your recovery programme. I understand that there might be a cost concern, but consider this: supplements and herbs can be quite pricey, and costs can quickly add up. and without a planned treatment programme, you might be cherry picking without any substantial results, and that is a great waste of money. Most therapists try their absolute best to keep prices affordable.

Herbal medicines which restore and support the adrenal glands

Miraculously, there are plants which can restore energy to the exhausted adrenal glands, and the fatigued mind and body. These herbs fall into the class of adaptogenic herbs, and while this is a fairly loosely defined term, essentially it refers to a plants which help us cope or adapt to stressful situations. These plants have traditionally been used to support our survival during difficult periods of life, for example Siberian ginseng (*Eleuthrococcus senticosus*) was used by the elderly folk in Russia to help them survive long and freezing winters with little food. Another example is *Sutherlandia frutescens* which the Zulus of South Africa call *"insiswa"*, meaning "to take away the darkness". This beautiful plant with red bubble-like seed pods was taken by the Zulu warriors after their wars when they returned exhausted and suffering from post-traumatic-stress-disorder, as we now know that soldiers often do.

In both of these examples, the plants helped men and women to cope and survive through either the stressful situation itself, or the effects that the stress had on the person's wellbeing. Our lives may not be as dramatic as either of these examples, but in many cases, the stress is long term and unrelenting. Our bodies cannot differentiate between what *type* of stress we are experiencing – just that we *are* experiencing stress and after some time the body has difficulty coping. This is when we need adaptogenic herbs, as well as the adrenal supporting herbs, calming herbs, excellent food, proper rest and kindness to ourselves.

Liquorice (*Glycyrrhiza glabra*)

Liquorice has long been used to help with the recovery of adrenal fatigue. In fact, it was once the "drug" of choice for the treatment of Addison's disease, which is a disease of complete adrenal failure. Liquorice root has natural constituents with cortisol-like effects, thus sparing the adrenal glands the necessity of producing its own cortisol steroid, and allowing the gland to rest and recover.

In accordance with steroid-like actions, liquorice demonstrates clear anti-inflammatory and anti-allergic actions.[1] Although there isn't a test to show this imbalance, the general picture of a poor ability to recover from viral infections, and excessive inflammatory and allergic reactions, will suggest Th1/Th2 immune imbalance. Marvellously, liquorice is not only a natural anti-inflammatory herb, but also has anti-viral properties.[2][3]

For these reasons, liquorice is an excellent choice for those who are burnt out with a poor immune response to viruses. There is a caution, however. Large doses of liquorice can increase the blood pressure and reduce potassium levels, and this herb should be avoided if you have high blood pressure or kidney disease. Although most people thrive on liquorice, it can make a tiny percentage more jittery, and they will need a gentler option for a while.

Chinese foxglove (*Rehmannia glutinosa*)

Rehmannia has been used in China for a very long time as a vitality tonic for those who suffer from weakness and anaemia. Like liquorice, it supports the adrenal glands, but this herb does not raise the blood pressure. Rehmannia root is cool, dark and sweet, and particularly indicated for those who feel physically weak with a sensation of too much heat or a great thirst. One very interesting study describes how rehmannia improves the immune system in those with yin deficiency.[4] In Chinese medicine, yin deficiency describes over-agitation with a lack of coolness and moisture.

I describe to my patients the effect of rehmannia as being a soft, sweet, cooling mist over a burning desert. But it does so much more than cool, it also has a fortifying, balancing and strengthening effect on the blood, the immune system, cardiovascular system, nervous system and endocrine system – really, on the whole body. I love to use it with Damascus rose, especially for menopausal women suffering from burnout.

Siberian ginseng (*Eleutherococcus senticosus*)

Siberian ginseng is a herb native to Russia, where it has been traditionally used to help elderly people survive long freezing winters with little food. These days, herbalists use it to support those who experience constant and unrelenting stress and depleted immunity. Siberian ginseng is both an adrenal and immune tonic, so this is a herb that I might consider for those who exhibit poor immunity such as recurrent colds from which they have difficulty recovering, but at the same time the person feels gravely fatigued. I see this herb as a very protective and strengthening herb, using it for those who feel weak and vulnerable to viruses, and especially winter ills.

Ashwagandha (*Withania somnifera*)

Ashwagandha comes from India, and according to Ayurvedic medicine, is classified as a *rasayana*, which refers to herbs which promote physical and mental health, improve resistance against disease and stress, and revitalize the body. In other words, ashwagandha is also an adaptogen. I absolutely love using this herb because it calms the mind and strengthens the body at the same time. I tell my patients that it is like compost in the soil – it nourishes you back to health. It is particularly helpful for people who have been debilitated for long periods of time, where they feel weak, jittery, easily succumbing to shock or fright with further weakness and fragility.

Usually, someone in that state has a very poor libido. Discussing libido may seem as if I am deviating from the point, but a person's libido is a good indication of their vitality or energy levels. If you are too tired or wired, sex isn't going to happen.

Hence, this ashwagandha herb restores energy levels in those who are debilitated, and is also used as a sexual and fertility tonic for those with stress-related infertility.[5]

Ashwagandha helps to rebalance the immune system when Th1 is too low,[6] and it is currently exciting attention among scientists as a herb with such powerful anti-viral actions that it "could be implicated in the management and treatment of flu and flu-like diseases connected with SARS-

CoV-2",[7] making it an excellent candidate not only for Long Covid and posti-viral fatigue, but also for adrenal burnout.

Withania is one of my favourite herbs to give at bedtime, because it aids sleep, whilst at the same time, helps to restore the adrenals overnight. Have a look at the name – *Withania somnifera*; Somnus was the Roman god of sleep. One of my favourite sleeping formulas to give to people is *Withania*, valerian, passionflower and liquorice. The ashwaganda, *Passiflora* and valerian allow you to let go and guide you into a deep sleep whilst the ashwagandha and liquorice nourish your adrenals whilst you sleep. Aren't plants just wonderful? They are like green angels.

Rose root *(Rhodiola rosea)*

Rose root grows at high altitudes, and traditionally has been given for strength and to protect against altitude sickness to those making mountain crossings. Consider the symptoms of altitude sickness – and note how similar they are to long-term stress induced fatigue: headache, nausea, extreme fatigue and weakness, dizziness, sleep disturbance, feelings of malaise, palpitations – and note how similar they are to long-term stress-induced fatigue.

I love to use rose root to support those who are suffering from emotional fatigue. This root supports our emotional response to stress, and has been shown to reduce cortisol secretion, thus helping to protect the adrenal glands from over work, and the rosy fragrance also has a comforting effect for emotional exhaustion.

Research has also shown that rose root can significantly relieve mild to moderate depression. One particular study compared rose root to sertraline and found that although the latter had the stronger effect, rose root had fewer side effects.[8]

This is a herb which can be used to support physical and mental resources, but as a medical herbalist treating stressed people under everyday conditions, I find rose root particularly good for people who are physically weakened as a result of emotional exhaustion, and thus feel utterly drained, fragile and debilitated.

Don't you find this intriguing? What business has a herb to do with a calming action, or an anti-depressant action? As far as we know, plants do not suffer from sadness or depression, so we can only conclude that these properties are there to support the human/animal kingdom. What a sacrifice plants make for us by offering their roots, their whole body, to restore us. With this in mind, we should take our herbal medicines with gratitude and awe at the magnificent benevolence of the plant kingdom.

Schizandra (*Schisandra chinensis*)

Schizandra grows in the far north of China and Russia. It is known as the five-flavour fruit because it is said to possess the five basic flavours, being simultaneously salty, sweet, sour, pungent and bitter. This herb is a classic adaptogen, effectively helping the body to cope well with stress by reducing cortisol and the effects of stress on the body. It is also a potent antioxidant herb, helping to reduce inflammation while at the same time supporting the liver through its detoxification processes. At the same time, it also increases stamina and reduces fatigue.

Traditional Chinese Medicine states the Qi (life force) fails to circulate through the body if the Liver is stagnant. You will notice that I write Liver with a capital L, because in Chinese medicine, the Liver does not represent the organs as we understand them in Western medicine. According to Traditional Chinese Medicine, the Liver circulates the Qi. However, when a person feels angry or frustrated over a period of time, these emotions congest the Liver, making it "stagnant". Now the Liver is unable to circulate the Qi, and so the person feels fatigued or devitalized. On the other hand, if the Liver is stagnant due to toxic build up, then frustration and anger may ensue – think how you feel in a traffic jam when you are trying to get somewhere.

Schizandra is a well-known liver tonic, and I use it as a refreshing and revitalizing herb for those who feel hot, sluggish and fatigued, and possibly irritable. I find it very helpful for women who are experiencing menopausal flushes and at the same time feel completely wrung out.

Gotu kola (Centella asiatica)

Gotu kola, also known as Indian or Asiatic pennywort, is a quiet herb, and one which I have valued for years in helping those who are burnt out mentally and have difficulty focusing their attention, holding a conversation, reading or even following a television story. Sometimes this symptom is so severe that a person will describe it as "brain ache", and may have a strong aversion to any sensory stimulation, often wishing to remain in a quiet and darkened room for extended periods of time. Gotu kola helps to restore normal brain function and has been used by the healers of India for this purpose for about 2,000 years.

Traditional medicine uses gotu kola to support the ageing brain, improve mood and cognition, and enhance memory. Scientific studies show this herb to be antioxidant, highly anti-inflammatory and possess nerve-regenerative properties. Furthermore, it inhibits nerve toxicity, reduces anxiety and depression. What a fabulous herb, and indeed, it is. I find that it works very quickly for people who feel mentally fatigued.[9]

One of the symptoms of adrenal fatigue is slow wound healing, and gotu kola can support the whole body because of its collagen-boosting effects. Collagen is the stuff which holds all our tissues together, and it is needed for the health of our body tissues,[10] otherwise we feel as if we are literally "falling apart".

Caterpillar fungus (*Cordyceps sinensis*)

This is a slightly sinister, truly fascinatingly mushroom. High on the Tibetan plateau at about 3,000m live certain species of caterpillar which becomes infected by a fungus. The fungus then proceeds to feed off the living caterpillar, eventually killing it, so that what is left is a thin, brown, reed-like mushroom growing out of the head of a mummified caterpillar.

About 1,500 years ago, the Tibetan herdsmen noticed that their animals became much stronger and more fortified after eating this fungus. Word spread to local doctors, and soon it became so highly regarded that there was a "fungal gold rush". Happily for caterpillars, these days the fungus is grown on agar in a laboratory, making it much more affordable but just as effective.

Caterpillar fungus (*Cordyceps*) has two major traditional properties. The first being has been shown to have anti-ageing effect, and its ability to enhancing athletic performance, and also improves low libido and increases fertility in both men and women. It is said to make old people feel young again. So you can imagine why it was such high in demand. As an anti-viral agent and immune modulator, caterpillar fungus is highly valuable for those with debilitating post-viral fatigue.

Sutherlandia (*Sutherlandia frutescens*)

Sutherlandia frutescens, also known as cancer bush, has been referred to as the African adaptogen *par excellence*, and it has a very strong tradition as a herb to take after a period of stress. The Zulus of South Africa call it *insiswa*, and Zulu warriors would take it when they returned from combat, exhausted and often suffering from post-traumatic stress disorder.

In terms of its effects on the adrenal glands, studies have shown that *Sutherlandia* showed a reduced cortisol response during periods of stress, and can alleviate depression in stressful situations.[11]

Like so many of the restorative herbs we have looked at, *Sutherlandia* shows antioxidant actions, which may also account for its traditional anti-inflammatory[12] and strengthening applications.

It is rich in amino acids L-canavanine and L-arginine, which have anti-viral properties, potentially against the Covid virus, and we see this effect reflected in its traditional use in Africa against HIV and the influenza virus.[13]

All these actions together suggest that *Sutherlandia* could be an almost perfect herb to use in stress-related illness, because it maintains normal cortisol levels, supports emotional health, is anti-inflammatory, is traditionally used to restore stamina and is an anti-viral herb.

Nutritional foods to nourish the adrenal glands

These are my four favourite nutritional supplements to support adrenal fatigue. For more in-depth nutritional support, please see a nutritionist or dietician.

Essential fatty acids

The reason they are called essential is because our body needs these fatty acids for good health but is unable to manufacture them, and therefore must aquire them from food. It is well known that our Western diet is high in omega-6 and lower in omega-3 fatty acids, but perhaps it is less well known that stress reduces the amount of omega-3 in our body. The interesting thing is that omega-3 fatty acids have been found to reduce the stress-induced cortisol spike, and thus moderate our response to stress. In this way, omega-3 fatty acids can support and preserve our adrenal function.

Foods rich in essential fatty acids include:

- Oily fish (mackerel, sardines, salmon, tuna steak)

- Walnuts

- Chia seeds

- Flaxseeds

- Algae oil.

B vitamins

Vitamin B is a class of vitamins which are largely concerned with providing energy to our cells, and supporting a healthy nervous system. Having sufficient vitamin B supports the function of a healthy heart, helps us to cope with stress, provides the necessary elements for good physical stamina, and enhances the quality of our skin and hair.

A vitamin B complex is my number one vitamin supplement that I will give those who are burned out, because the body is crying out for the nutrition needed to support the nervous system. People can be so exhausted that they feel as if they are trembling on the inside, their hair is falling out, their skin has lost its glow, and they can't seem to relax. A vitamin B complex will really help to fortify the nervous system, support your energy and reduce anxiety, stress responses and depression.

Foods rich in B vitamins include:

- Oats

- Nuts

- Organ meats

- Egg yolks

- Wholegrain bread

- Berries

- Brown rice

- Soya beans

- Black strap molasses.

Vitamin C

Vitamin C is not only essential for our immune response, but also aids the absorption of iron, and helps to synthesize some of the adrenal hormones, as well as progesterone and testosterone. Vitamin C gets burned up when we are stressed out. The problem is that it is a water-soluble vitamin, but our cell walls are made up of a fatty membrane known as the phospholipid bilayer (more on which later). Since fats repel water, a large proportion of ordinary vitamin C that we get from food is excreted in the urine.

Liposomal vitamin C, however, has been packaged into tiny fat droplets, which are easily able to slip through the cell membrane into the interior of the cell. It is more expensive, but it is also significantly better absorbed.

Having said all this, I love food state vitamins. During World War II, children were paid to pick rosehips, which were manufactured on a large scale into a vitamin C rich syrup to support the immunity of the children. For us, it is a lovely late-summer ritual to spend an afternoon wandering down the hedgerows, collecting wild rosehips, and then taking them home to make into a winter tonic for you and your family.

Foods rich in vitamin C include:

- Red peppers

- Tomatoes

- Strawberries

- Papaya

- Pink grapefruit

- Broccoli.

Magnesium

Magnesium is one of the most important minerals for your adrenal glands, providing the necessary energy for your adrenals – and every cell in your body for that matter – to function properly. It is also a fabulous muscle relaxant for jumpy legs, or that horrible, exhausted-but-can't-switch-off feeling. Sometimes, if I am struggling to sleep, I will take a magnesium capsule and 5ml of valerian tincture, and before I know it, I am sound asleep.

Foods rich in magnesium include:

- Oats

- Pumpkin seeds

- Cashew nuts

- Brown rice

- Avocado

- Spinach.

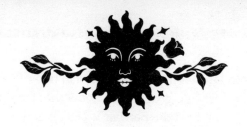

CHAPTER 8

POST-VIRAL FATIGUE AND LONG COVID

So far in this book we have discovered the profound impact stress has on the adrenal glands, forcing them to release higher levels of cortisol than is sustainable while we attempt to navigate our hectic modern-day lifestyles. We have seen how, over time, this depresses the anti-viral arm of the immune system (Th1), meaning we are more susceptible to viral infections which don't resolve, such as post-viral fatigue syndrome, and also elevates the allergic arm of the immune system (Th2), which means we are more vulnerable to inflammatory and some autoimmune conditions such as rheumatoid arthritis.[1]

It is like an accident waiting to happen, whereby the mind–body system is just hanging on the edge with stress, either due to a major life event, or ongoing life events over the years, or even chemical stressors such as long-term exposure to environmental toxins like black mould and mycoplasmas. Then the final straw, being a viral infection, plummets the person over the edge.

Glandular fever

A frequent cause of ongoing deep fatigue is post-viral fatigue, often as a result of glandular fever, and now, Long Covid. Glandular fever is most commonly seen in younger people in their mid- to late teens up until the mid-twenties, although it can occur in all age groups. We know that glandular fever is caused by the Epstein–Barr virus (EBV), and while EBV is referred to as the underlying cause, I have to ask: why don't the parents of those young people with glandular fever get ill? Or their classmates for that matter?

Those young people who catch EBV and then develop glandular fever are often fit and healthy, and yet I often find that they were going through a particularly stressful time in their life when they contracted the virus. Perhaps they have been studying for exams, or there are difficulties at home. Quite often, I have noticed, a beloved grandparent or family pet may have died a few months or even a year or two before they became ill. Although these are seen as normal life events, adolescence is invariably a very stressful time in one's life. When we consider the added stresses of getting good enough grades to get to university,[2] constant news feeds, the pressures surrounding social media and the climate crisis, young people are actually under tremendous strain, and it is not surprising that their immune systems may be compromised.

Then the Epstein–Barr virus comes along, and bang – glandular fever. Unbelievably, they are often prescribed antibiotics (for a virus), which is completely useless, and those antibiotics kill not only infectious bacteria, but the gut microbes, which significantly disrupts the immune system, pushing the person further towards Th2 domination and being less able to fight off the viral attack.[3]

When I have a young patient with glandular fever, I consider it a case of great urgency, because if that virus takes hold, it can quite easily develop into post-viral fatigue. I prescribe anti-viral herbs as soon as possible, with immune tonics, probiotics and glandular cleansers. If necessary, I also recommend adrenal herbs, as well as rest, rest, rest, until they are better. Usually, the young person responds quickly, the crisis passes, and they can get on with their lives.

But what about those people who did not recover, and who go on to develop post-viral fatigue or Long Covid? Recovery can be made, but it is a slower process.

Long Covid

Long Covid is defined as remaining sick for three months or more after the initial SARS-CoV-2 infection, and as we all know, it has affected a lot of people – more than 17 million in just the first two years of the pandemic, according to the World Health Organization.[4]

One might argue that Long Covid was definitely caused by a virus, and is therefore not related to stress, and that is true – there was certainly a very nasty novel virus. However, we must remember that at the time of the pandemic, there was mass panic. All we ever heard on the news was that millions were going to die, and that millions *were* dying.

I remember my patients being terrified, living in a state of perpetual upset, and I spent most of my consultations calming people down. Then everyone was confined to their homes and unable to visit their loved ones. Grandparents were banned from hugging their grandchildren and people died alone in hospital from all sorts of problems, but they died isolated from their family who were not allowed to visit them. People lost their businesses and their incomes, and then there was the huge issue between pro- and anti-vaxxers. Families were torn apart. It was like a societal and psychological Armageddon, the repercussions of which will be felt for years to come. I for one wonder what this stress did to the immune systems of the human population.

During World War II, there was a government campaign which actively encouraged people to collect rosehips and make vitamin C rich syrup as an immune tonic, but 80 years later, our governments were are too smart for that – we all had to be vaccinated, and not a word about vitamin C, vitamin D or rosehips issued on the news bulletins.

So here we have it – a mass panic with long-term stress which depresses the immune response to viral infection but increases allergic response, not many people using immune-supportive natural remedies, and then a nasty viral trigger.

Neuro-inflammation (brain in flames)

There is growing evidence that people with chronic fatigue syndrome and Long Covid have widespread neuro-inflammation in the brain.[5] The viral infection triggers the immune system to mobilize inflammatory cells in the brain as a protective response. Just like the leaky gut wall, the fine membrane (known as the blood–brain barrier), which usually protects the brain from toxic damage, becomes more permeable, thus allowing the inflammatory molecules and toxins to enter the brain and set up an inflammatory response.[6] This is called neuro-inflammation, and it is like the brain is on fire. It is a big problem and very disruptive to the body.

The inflammation in the brain has far-reaching consequences for the person because the brain and spinal cord constitutes the central nervous system, which is the conductor of information to and from every cell in the body. So many of the seemingly weird symptoms related to this disease can be traced to inflammation in the central nervous system: changes in mood, loss of temperature control, irregular blood pressure, dizziness, difficulty concentrating, sleep disturbances. Even the joint and muscle pain can be the result of the brain triggering pain sensations. The neuro-inflammation also affects the cranial nerves in the brain, resulting in loss of taste and smell, an altered voice, and sometimes nausea.

If the underlying stress is not resolved, the inflammation becomes chronic (ongoing), resulting in the breakdown of the homeostatic balance within the entire system of the body.[7] I feel that it is important to underline here, that the scientists of these studies refer to stressful events as being psychological, environmental (possibly prolonged exposure to moulds and mycotoxins or heavy metals), physical (such as an accident or major surgery), or it could be a viral infection. In the case of post-viral illness, it may be that the current stress is a hidden reservoir of viruses perpetuating the illness. Whatever form it takes, the underlying cause must be addressed.

If the initial stressor is not resolved, the inflammatory molecules (called cytokines) cause ongoing neuro-inflammation, which continues to disrupt the homeostatic balance of the body, affecting all the body systems in a vicious cycle where the disruption stimulates the inflammation, which further disrupts the homeostatic balance. This perpetuates the post-viral fatigue of CFS and Long Covid, and even allows for more serious relapses. Once the homeostatic balance has been disrupted, the person finds it difficult to recover from the normal life activities that they were able to do previously, and thus, for example, they become very tired after a small outing, sometimes taking days to recover.

Inflammation is widespread. A common symptom such as shortness of breath is not caused by spasms of the bronchi, as in asthma, but is called "air-hunger", the result of the chronic inflammation in the lung tissue.[8] When the body tissues are inflamed for an extended period of time, the inflamed tissues harden into leathery scar tissue called fibrosis, which is much less flexible than healthy lung tissues, and consequently the person finds it difficult to get enough air.

The Th1/Th2 disturbance, where the anti-viral arm of the immune system is lowered but the allergic inflammatory arm is raised, can account for the allergic symptoms such as skin hives, and the sudden increase in people suffering with histamine intolerance, and mast cell activation syndrome (MCAS) that we are seeing.

The SARS-CoV-2 virus initiated a widespread inflammation of the inside lining of the blood vessels called the endothelium,[9] which bleed and form micro-clots – massively damaging to the organs of the body, especially the lungs, heart, kidneys and the brain. Long Covid symptoms, specifically fatigue and chest pain, are associated with this ongoing endothelial damage.[10]

The SARS-CoV-2 virus is particularly harsh in that it reactivates viruses which were dormant in the body. Herpes viruses, the Epstein–Barr virus, the varicella zoster virus (shingles) and cytomegalovirus are reactivated by Covid, overwhelming the body with a cascade of immune inflammatory chemicals.

When dealing with Long Covid or any post-viral illness, we have to ask the question: are we dealing with a live virus, or the damage done by the virus? How do we assess that?

The way I do that in my practice is that if my patient tells me that they have recurrent fever, enlarged glands, night sweats and flu-like symptoms, I assume that there is an ongoing or reactivated viral presence, and I use strong anti-viral herbs, and particularly, herbs to strengthen the immune system against the attackers.

As I write, there is no definitive diagnostic test for Long Covid or post-viral fatigue syndrome, just as there isn't one for chronic fatigue syndrome/ME. The diagnosis is made by your health practitioner through a clinical assessment and is based on a symptom pattern which matches that of common symptoms associated with Long Covid or post-viral fatigue syndrome. To be diagnosed, symptoms must have also been preceded by a viral infection, and continued for longer than three months. Your doctor may run several tests to rule out other long-term illnesses.

In terms of the symptom list, this is a blurry subject, because Long Covid is a form of post-viral fatigue, yet there are differences, which you will see in the two lists below. It is important to note that not everyone will have all of the symptoms listed.

Symptoms of Long Covid

- Overwhelming fatigue and weakness

- Ongoing fever

- General feeling of malaise

- Breathlessness

- Recurrent cough/sore throat

- Chest pain/tightness

- Dizziness, light-headedness and palpitations upon standing, known as PoTS (postural tachycardia syndrome)

- Brain fog

- Loss of concentration

- Poor memory

- Frequent headaches

- Disturbed sleep

- Pins and needles, and numbness in fingers and toes

- Sudden confusion (delirium), particularly in older people

- Changes to eyesight

- Shingles

- Abdominal pain

- Nausea

- Ongoing diarrhoea

- Weak and/or painful muscles

- Aching joints

- Low mood and depression

- Anxiety

- Loss of taste and/or smell

- Tinnitus

- Skin rashes, or extreme skin sensitivity

- Hair loss.

Symptons of post-viral fatigue syndrome

- Profound and ongoing fatigue which is not relieved by sleep

- General feeling of malaise

- Frequent or ongoing headaches

- Nausea

- Stomach cramps

- Difficulty digesting food

- Muscle pain

- Fibromyalgia

- Joint pains

- Low mood

- Sleep difficulties

- Poor concentration

- Difficulty finding words

- Difficulty focusing

- Brain fog

- Frequent sore throat

- Frequent enlarged glands

- General flu-like symptoms.

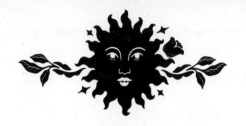

CHAPTER 9

REPAIR YOUR MITOCHONDRIA

Thus far we have looked at how chronic fatigue affects the immune system and the adrenal glands as a result of either long-term stress or a severe shock. However, stress also affects the very inner workings of our cells.

The powerhouses of the cell

Each of the 50 trillion cells in your body looks a bit like a fried egg. The yolk represents the nucleus of the cell, and within the white of the fried egg, there are other little bubbles called organelles, which all have different jobs to do. Some are called mitochondria, and they produce our energy. Of all the organs in our body, the brain carries by far the highest number of mitochondria.

The mitochondria are commonly referred to as the powerhouses of our cells. You might think of them as little factories, with a system of cogs and wheels that together make up what's called the Krebs Cycle, which spits out packets of energy called ATP (adenosine triphosphate). This is our energy currency. If you have abundant ATP, you have abundant energy, but if your mitochondria are damaged, then you have too little energy and it takes a long time to recover from anything which requires energy output. Everything in life, even thinking, requires energy, so when the mitochondria are damaged, that person is always in energy deficit.

Just like money, when you spend it, more needs to be generated. So these ATP packets of energy have to be replenished constantly. Usually this is something we don't even think about. If we feel a little tired, we take a rest, and then we regain our energy, but for people who are chronically fatigued, it can take days to recover their energy levels from even the mildest exertion. Even then, their energy levels are way below par. These people need far more time than healthy people do, to replace the spent energy packets.

Thus, clearly, a person with constant fatigue has damaged mitochondria, but the big question in my mind has always been – So, how do the mitochondria in those people with chronic fatigue become so damaged in the first place? If we can understand this, perhaps we have an opportunity to repair that damage and bring the person back to full health.

Studies have shown that psychological stress, such as adverse childhood events, discrimination, job strain, emotional trauma, the pressures of care giving and social isolation can all damage our mitochondria.[1] Long-term stress increases inflammatory molecules, which makes the mitochondria swell, thereby distending and damaging the surrounding mitochondrial membrane. As a result, this damage decreases energy production capacity[2] while speeding up the ageing process inside the cells. This in turn increases the risk of disease.[3]

A highly respected hypothesis comes from Martin L. Pall, a professor emeritus of biochemistry and basic medical sciences at Washington State University, specializing in chronic fatigue syndrome. In his book *Explaining Unexplained Illness*, he outlines a detailed proposal for the mechanism by which the mitochondria become damaged.

Linking psychological stress (as well as other stresses such as viral infection, physical trauma and toxic accumulations, among others) to a little-known cycle referred to as NO/ONOO (pronounced "no oh no"), he describes how prolonged or severe stress significantly increases the production of a chemical called nitric oxide (NO). Nitric oxide, in turn, ratchets up a chemical called peroxynitrite (ONOO), which stimulates oxidative damage within the cell, and then back loops to re-stimulate the nitric oxide again – creating a vicious cycle of inflammation and damage. We have already discussed how cortisol reduces inflammation, and yet if someone has fatigued adrenal glands, they cannot produce the cortisol needed to control the inflammatory process, and so the net effect is oxidative damage to the cells and mitochondria.

The mitochondria are encased in a fatty membrane known as a phospholipid bilayer, and when this is ruptured, it leaks the packets of ATP energy, which, as you can imagine, is a disaster. The good news, however, is that this information tells us that antioxidants and phospholipid therapy can be very useful tools to use in the recovery process, and in fact, one of the major routes to recovery which is being discovered for Long Covid is antioxidant therapy.

So, now we see that psychological or long-term day-to-day stress can damage the mitochondria, but what this has to do with post-viral fatigue?

Mitochondria have their own DNA and RNA, which replicates independently of the DNA and RNA in the nucleus of the cell.[4] During viral infections, the virus directly targets the mitochondria and hijacks its RNA or DNA for its own reproduction. But then the virus goes even further by cleverly disabling the natural anti-viral responses. The result is that the body's energy production is damaged, we can't think clearly because the mitochondria in our brain which share information are profoundly injured, and, of course, the person is more vulnerable than ever to further viral insult.

Widespread environmental toxins such as micro-plastics, heavy metals like mercury, lead and arsenic, and pesticides are all known to damage the mitochondria of our cells.[5] [6] Even common medicines such as sertraline, beta blockers and aspirin have mitochondrial toxicity as an unintended side effect.[7]

The typical Western diet can also be extremely damaging to our mitochondria. As study even found that female mice who were fed a high-sugar/high-fat diet not only developed mitochondrial dysfunction, but this trait was passed down to their offspring through three generations, despite the diet being corrected.[8]

It is a sad fact of life that we live in a very toxic world. As such, we have no choice but to consider the effects of environmental toxins, because they are also major disruptors of mitochondrial health. Thankfully, humans are waking up to the environmental disaster which affects every living being on this earth, but we do not yet live in a clean world, and so moving away from these environmental toxins is necessary to help your mitochondrial recovery.

Below is just a very short list of some common foods in which mitochondrial toxins are very commonly found:

- Transfats – found in fried fast foods, certain pies, burgers, sausage rolls and margarine

- Mercury – found in dental fillings, seafoods such as tuna and sword fish, and sea salt

- Lead – found in chocolate, peas, apple and grape juice

- Arsenic – found in leafy vegetables and rice grown on soils which were previously treated with arsenic poisons.

It is widely accepted within the scientific community that in both chronic fatigue syndrome and Long Covid, the mitochondria are damaged, but a fascinating study released in December 2022 surmised that Long Covid may be the result of *prior* sub-optimal mitochondrial function. This suggests that the mitochondria were damaged *before* the viral infection, and Covid was the last straw, if you will, which toppled the person into a new inflammatory state from which they were unable to restore their healthy mitochondrial function, and thus their energy levels.

The paper suggests that prior mitochondrial health is necessary for resistance to the Covid virus,[9] and if we expand on that – why not other viruses too, such as the Epstein–Barr virus associated with glandular fever?

This may all sound pretty bleak, but the good news is that the body has remarkable powers of regeneration and recovery – as long as we provide the correct environment and necessary building materials. I personally have seen many people recover from long-term fatigue, so it can be done.

Healing the mitochondria

Before we can even think of repairing the mitochondria, environmental toxins need to be removed from our cells. This is not an easy job, I grant you, because there are man-made toxins in the water, soil and air, but we can do a lot to counter these negative influences on our heath, and plants can be our ally in this.

Above all, do not harm.

Interestingly, some of the traditionally most despised plants are actually our greatest unsung heroes. Nettles, pond slime (chlorella and spirulina), burdock and even clay can rescue us from our toxic burden. A deep detox, known as heavy metal chelation, is a tricky business, however, and I strongly recommend that you seek the guidance of someone professionally adept at this therapy if you feel that you need this level of detoxification.

Nonetheless, I am going to give you a detox programme which is both safe and effective.

Harness the power of plants

You can make a delightful start by filling your home with common houseplants. NASA conducted a study on the effects of plants on indoor pollutants, and the spider plant won the day by absorbing a whopping 95% of the pollutants tested. All plants will absorb toxins to a greater or lesser degree, as well as killing any wandering bacteria and moulds, all the while producing oxygen.[10]

Supermarkets often sell houseplants, but for some strange reason, they don't water them, and often I see sad nearly-dead plants which I love to rescue and give them a decent life. Plants bring a wonderful life force into a home, and by filling your home with indoor plants, you can change the energy of your home, and clean the air that you breathe.

Detoxifying herbs

When we detoxify the body, we go right inside the cells of the body. Herbs pull the toxins out of the cells and into the fluid between the cells, then the blood picks up the toxins and whooshes them away to the liver and kidneys where they are washed out of the body. In the liver, the toxins are broken down and flushed into the bowel, where they are evacuated with the faeces.

Liver and bowel support is therefore absolutely crucial, because if the liver is sluggish and over-burdened, or the bowel is congested, the toxins cannot be efficiently broken down and removed. Instead, there is a back-up of toxins in the blood which can actually cause the body significant harm. People who go through a detox can feel fatigued, have headaches, spotty skin, skin rashes, nausea, muscle pains and bad breath.

Thus, it is essential that the bowel is emptying at least once a day (preferably twice) so that the toxins flushed from the liver into the bowel are passed out of the body quickly.

So with a detox, we have to work backwards from the bowel to the cells. You start by making sure that your bowel is opening at least once a day, preferably twice. Below is an easy remedy to help to capture the toxins which have been flushed out of the liver, bulk up the stool and thereby stimulate a full and easy bowel movement.

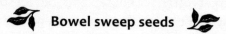 **Bowel sweep seeds**

Combine 2 dessertspoons of flaxseeds with half a cup of live plain yoghurt and eat with a bit of fruit if you wish. Follow this up with a large glass of water and within a day or two, you should experience very easy bowel movements and feel light and clean after going to the loo.

Now that the bowel is moving, you can think about encouraging the liver to flush the bile and toxins into the bowel. Herbs such as dandelion root, milk thistle, turmeric, ginger and lemon all encourage liver flushing.

At the same time, support kidney cleansing by eating foods like cucumber, celery and asparagus, and drinking dandelion leaf and nettle tea.

Now we move to the cells. Nettles are going to be our safe cellular detox agent, because they have the ability to remove heavy metals from the soil.[11] Herbalists have always used nettles to purify the blood, scavenge free radicals, as well as to build healthy blood cells thanks to nettles' diuretic actions and high mineral content. Nettles are not only cleansing and highly nutritious, but they are freely available and fun to collect, too. Just go out in the spring and harvest basketsful of fresh nettles from a clean area. If nettles grow in your garden, you can even cultivate a little patch by doing the "cut and come again" salad leaf method. Use them fresh, or dry and keep for later in the year. All you need to do is drop a sprig into a cup of boiling water and drink. You can also make nettle soups, nettle omelettes, nettle pesto – if you like to cook, you can really be creative with nettles.

Other foods which bind and eliminate the heavy metals include coriander (cilantro), garlic, organic blueberries, barley grass juice, black cherries, grapefruit, turmeric, onions, tomatoes, capers and radishes,[12] and these can be generously included in your diet.

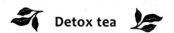 **Detox tea**

Put 3 sprigs of nettles (each about 6 leaves), – to remove the toxins from the cells
 5 slices of ginger, 2 slices of lemon and 4 dandelion leaves in a cup of boiling water and enjoy.

A gentle detox programme

1. First thing in the morning, drink a cup of Detox Tea (see above).

2. At some time during the day, eat your Bowel Sweep Seeds (see page 116), and immediately follow this with another large cup of Detox Tea.

3. Drink plenty of water during the day to wash the toxins out of the bloodstream into the kidneys and liver. If you add a pinch of chilli powder, the effect will be even stronger.

4. Have a hot Epsom salt bath or sauna for about 20 minutes, three times a week. Make sure that you rinse the sweat off your skin before you get dressed. (If you

are very weak or struggle with dizziness or low blood pressure, you can skip this step.)

5. Start your cleansing programme gently with one cup of Detox Tea daily, then after three days take two cups daily, and another three days later, you can take three cups daily. You can continue with up to three cups daily for three months.

Antioxidant-rich foods

As I mentioned earlier, the mitochondria are encased in a membrane called the phospholipid bilayer, and as the free radicals crash around, tearing holes in the phospholipid membrane, the energy packets of ATP spill out, leaving that person energy deficient. Plants come to the rescue once again as you fill your plate with antioxidants to mop up those free radicals and neutralize their damaging effect.

There are plenty of antioxidant products on the market and just looking at the vast array can be overwhelming, but you can go a long way towards healing yourself by eating a diet rich in antioxidants. There is so much that

Let food be your medicine.

can be done with diet to improve one's health, and this is wonderfully empowering because it puts your health back into your own hands.

For those who are terribly fatigued, this can be a moot point, because they can barely manage to go shopping for food, let alone cook a fantastic meal. Perhaps you can recruit friends and family members to rally around and help you a little, until you have restored your health to the point where you can feel enthusiastic about cooking healthy meals for yourself. Alternatively, yourself or someone else can cook in greater quantities, then divide into portions and freeze.

With regards diet, you need to be strict about junk food so that you are not ingesting poisons. The deep fried fast food junk food is full full full of damaging substances which increase the free radical and toxic load on your cells, interfere with your hormones, and clog up the detoxification pathways of the cells and the liver. Just watch the YouTube film "Supersize Me" to get an idea how badly junk food will affect your health. There are so many luscious healthy foods to be enjoyed instead.

The Rainbow Diet

The Rainbow Diet is one which incorporates all the different colours of vegetables into your diet: red, orange, yellow, green, blue, indigo and violet. Foods with a variety of colours, as these will be loaded with a whole range of healthy nutrients: vitamins, minerals, microelements, all bursting with antioxidants.

Spinach and Swiss chard – peppers, red, yellow and green – aubergine – tomatoes – red cabbage – asparagus – cranberries – blackberries – blueberries – strawberries – sweet potato – raspberries – red grapes – lemons and grapefruit – beetroot – buckwheat – fresh rosemary – fresh thyme – fresh basil – fresh peppermint – dark chocolate – red wine – olive oil – sesame seeds (tahini) – alfalfa and bean sprouts

Take a look at the fantastic variety of anti-oxidants in common foods:

• Sweet potato – contains beta carotene

- Artichokes – contain rutin, quercetin, silymarin, and gallic acid

- Red peppers – contain carotenoids

- Blueberries, blackberries, raspberries, strawberries, goji berries – contain anthocyanins and anthocyanidins

- Walnuts and pecans – contain polyphenols

- Kale – contains beta-carotene, and vitamins C and E

- Dark chocolate – contains flavonoids

- Garlic – contains allicin

- Tomatoes – contains lycopene

- Red cabbage – contains anthocyanins

- Beans such as broad beans – contain kaempferol

- Beetroot – contains betalains

- Spinach – contains lutein and zeaxanthin.

And here are some common kitchen condiments with antioxidant actions:

Turmeric root (*Curcuma longa*)

Turmeric exerts significant anti-oxidant effects on cells, and the excellent thing about turmeric is that it is lipophilic (fat loving), thus it can cross the phospholipid bilayer into the cell, and importantly, it can cross into the inflamed central nervous system. This Indian root is well known to exert significant antioxidant and anti-inflammatory actions on these important cells, and thereby helps to restore mitochondrial function. Herbalists love this natural medicine for the above action and also because it is a liver-supporting herb, which is so important when we initiate the detoxification programme.

The so-called active ingredient in turmeric is curcumin, but the problem is that curcumin is very poorly available to the cells because it is poorly absorbed by the intestines and the cells. This is because it is not water soluble, but fat soluble. The Indian grandmothers used to cook turmeric spice gently with ghee and a grind of black pepper as a cure for many illnesses. They knew what they were doing, because the buttery ghee is attractive to the fat-loving curcumin and helps to transport it across the digestive wall into the blood whilst the black pepper prevents it breakdown, therefore keeping the curcumin available for the cells for longer. The fat/ghee (or coconut oil) combination also facilitates the curcumin crossing into the brain where it cools the inflammation whilst helping to restore mitochondria in the brain.[13] [14]

Sesame seeds

Tahini is a seed butter made entirely from crushed sesame seeds and is a powerful food medicine. Sesame seeds are highly anti-oxidant, and have been shown to protect the brain from anti-oxidant damage and neuro-degenerative diseases such as dementia. It is not hard to extrapolate this to the brain-fog of all forms of fatigue.

Rosemary (*Rosmarinus officinalis*)

Rosemary is a beloved garden plant and well established as a traditional remedy for improving circulation and gladdening the heart. Indeed, if you rub your hand over the plant, the fragrance which floats towards your nose does indeed gladden the heart.

For our discussion, it is worth noting that rosemary has significant anti-oxidant properties, quenching the free radicals in the mitochondria, thus protecting your energy factories against damage. It also liver protective, supporting the detoxification process which is necessary to unclog the mitochondria from harmful toxic debris.

Rosemary is perhaps best known for its ability to improve circulation and memory. By relaxing the blood vessels and slightly thinning the blood, more valuable nutrients can be delivered to the cells, whilst at the same time transporting cellular toxins away to be processed in the liver.

Ginger (*Zingiber officinalis*)

Ordinary kitchen ginger is a powerful anti-oxidant, anti-viral and has liver-supporting properties, but perhaps less well known is that this common spice can increase mitochondrial numbers and improve mitochondrial function.[15] In fact, the scientists of this study were so impressed with the herb, that they propose that ginger can be developed into a new remedy for mitochondrial dysfunction disorder. But we don't have to wait for that, because ginger is readily available in our grocery shops. I love to include ginger in my herbal prescriptions. When people are very fatigued and ill, I see an image of a camp fire which has gone cold, with only a tiny spark of warmth left. The person that I am sitting with feels cold and burned out, so I include ginger in my prescription to bring the warmth and life back to the cells.

Below is a warming and joyful tea with anti-oxidant, mitochondrial restorative, liver supporting, anti-microbial and circulatory stimulating properties. More than that, it is delicious and very comforting. I love to use this tea for those who are so debilitated, that they do not even have the energy to digest their food. This tea warms the stomach and helps to support digestion.

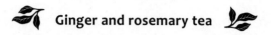

Ginger and rosemary tea

*Add a sprig of rosemary, 5 slices of fresh ginger
root, and a slice of lemon to a cup of boiling water.
Sweeten with a little honey if you wish. Drink two to
three times a day.*

Now that the cells are being relieved of their toxic burden, you can introduce foods which provide the building blocks to repair the mitochondrial membrane.

The mitochondrial wall is made of phospholipids, and so we should include foods rich in these molecules, such as eggs, fish, fish roe (fish eggs), soya beans, sunflower seeds, beef, pork and chicken. Eggs and fish are particularly rich in phospholipids, and fish roe (fish eggs) is very rich in phospholipids. For instance, whereas fish contains between 1–1.5% phospholipids, fish roe from herring, salmon and pollock contain between 38% and 75% of their lipids in the form of phospholipids.

Urolithin

The mighty oak is a very special and interesting tree. Wherever it grows in the world, it is a respected tree, valued for its strength, resilience and stability. Despite these qualities, its medical properties seemed (to me) to be strangely limited to the astringent actions of the tannins found in the leaves and bark. Until one day I happened upon this snippet of information, which I was able to follow up and discovered that the inner wood of oak heals and restores mitochondria!

Within the inner wood of the oak tree are compounds called roburins. Once in the intestine, our gut bacteria transform this into urolithin A and urolithin B. Amazingly, the urolithin levels seem to increase the gut bacteria responsible for the urolithin production.

Within the cell, urolithin A collects the damaged mitochondria and packs them off to the lysosomes, which break down damaged mitochondria and clear out cell debris and dead bacteria, and then reassemble the parts into perfectly healthy new mitochondria.

Urolithin B, in the meantime, increases muscle growth, and strength in the muscles, as well as helping those with erectile dysfunction. These appear to be testosterone effects, but if fact occurs without increasing testosterone levels.

Furthermore, the roburins possess potent antioxidant and free-radical scavenging properties, as well as anti-inflammatory and antithrombotic actions, which as we all know is part of the Long Covid picture.

The oak is shown to offer even more to our stressed-out, burned-out society. One of the worst effects of chronic fatigue is the difficulty in sleeping. Oak improves mood and sleep, decreases fatigue symptoms, enhances recovery from viral illnesses and the trauma of surgery. No side effects have been noted thus far, and bear in mind that humans have been maturing wine in oak for hundreds of years. This tree medicine is absolutely appropriate for post-traumatic stress disorder, post-viral fatigue, supporting the heart in mild heart failure and emotional fatigue

I make tinctures of oak and love to combine it in a prescription with other tinctures specific to each person's requirement, but you can also eat urolithin-rich foods, such as pomegranate, strawberries, blackberries, raspberries, walnuts, almonds, chestnuts, pistachios, pecans and tea.

And for those of you who enjoy a glass of wine: you can take the roburins in their original form if you drink red wine that has been aged in French oak barrels.

There is a caveat: roburins (only found in oak) and ellagic acid (berries and some nuts) are converted into urolithin A in the gut by rather obscure bacteria called *Gordonibacter pamelaeae* and *Bifidobacterium pseudocatenulatum*, which not everyone has and which you don't normally find in probiotic supplements. So the problem is that not everybody is able to convert these compounds into urolithins. This can be overcome by directly supplementing with urolithin A products, but these are very expensive, and ultimately, you need to produce your own urolithins.

As you have seen throughout this book, a healthy gut microbiome is central to your health, and those with the widest variety of friendly bacteria will be able to make the conversion. My suggestion is that you provide your body with the building blocks by eating lots of probiotic foods such as kefir, kimchi and sauerkraut. Then eat the prebiotic foods which feed these bacteria, such as onions, garlic, asparagus, banana, starchy root vegetables, as well as organic butter from grass-fed cows. Really up your intake in the foods which I list below.

Food sources of urolithin A:

Pomegranate – Strawberries – Blackberries – Raspberries – Walnuts – Almonds – Chestnuts – Pistachios – Pecans – Tea

This programme will reduce inflammation through your whole body, rebalance your immune system, heal your gut lining, enhance the conversations between the intestinal bacteria and the brain, and your microbiome and the mitochondria. It provides whole-body healing rather than just supplementing with urolithins, because the mitochondria are not damaged in isolation, they are damaged due to a lifestyle, and a final insult to the body which tipped you over the edge.

Honour yourself

As I write, I am working with several patients all with chronic fatigue, and they all have vastly different prescriptions of herbs, and yet my lifestyle advice to them is similar. To prescribe effectively, I have to get to know them. My patient and I form a relationship so that together we work out what triggered their particular fatigue, and then with herbs specific for each person, I am absolutely thrilled to see their health improving quite rapidly. But the advice that I give to all my patients is much the same as I am giving you in this book. Look after yourself, eat nourishing food, take the time to honour your body by resting because you cannot bust your way out of this illness.

I spoke to a lady yesterday, who said that she has come to realize that her ME gave her a huge gift. She had to face certain issues in the past, and then change who she was, to become more of the real her. A young man told me the same thing yesterday. He has to take off the people-pleasing mask that he has worn all his life to find out who he really is. It is scary but you cannot go back to being the same person that you were before, because that is why you ended up here. You have to connect with who you really are and then honour yourself. This takes time and the fatigue and rest that is enforced upon you allows you time to reflect. Please do hold yourself in love, because this is the environment in which you will heal.

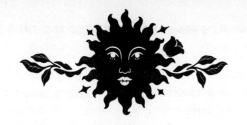

CHAPTER 10

HEALING HERBS FOR POST-VIRAL FATIGUE

The big question with Long Covid is: what is actually happening in the body? There appears to be three things that may be going on, but research at the time of writing this book has mainly focused on acute Covid, not Long Covid. However, there are three proposals, although the scientists suggest that it is likely that all three (and there are probably more) may work together to perpetuate this tragic illness.[1]

1. A persistent virus

2. A severely disrupted immune system leading to massive inflammation throughout the whole body

3. Damaged blood vessels leading to micro-clotting in the lungs, brain and other organs.

Let's consider what can be done, because it is important to tread very carefully with Long Covid on account of the massive inflammation which is caused by the disrupted immune system. If I briefly recap, Long Covid might be predicted by previously damaged mitochondria which could have been caused by stress. Long-term stress almost inevitably tips the immune balance from the healthy daily swing between Th1 and Th2, to being stuck in Th2 domination, which means that the body's ability to fight viral infection is compromised whilst being more predisposed towards inflammation, and allergic or some autoimmune conditions, thyroid disorders or rheumatoid arthritis.

Therefore, rather than stimulating the immune system, we want to rebalance it. As you can see from the theme of this book, this unfortunate body system is so over-stimulated that the person's health has collapsed. I prefer to nourish the immune system back to health, whilst at the same time, providing anti-viral herbs to kill the lingering viruses. There are many anti-viral herbs. Some are very strong and can be used with guidance from a medical herbalist. However, since this is a self-help book, I would like to introduce you to the benefits of herbs which are splendid options, many of which I would use in my prescriptions, but are safe and easily available in your kitchen or garden.

Bear in mind that the immune system starts in the gut, so it is important that you have adopted a diet with a wide range of colourful vegetables, as well as healthy proteins and fats. Besides providing antioxidants and nutrients, these colourful vegetables are rich in fibre, helping to move the bowels, cleansing out old toxic faecal matter as well as providing pre-biotics – the food for the friendly bacteria.

Strategy for recovery from post-viral fatigue:

• Seed the gut with friendly probiotics.

• Kill the viruses hiding in your tissues.

• Strengthen the immune system against viral attack.

• Rebalance the disrupted immune system.

• Heal the damaged blood vessels.

• Cool the inflammation.

Probiotics

It is interesting that as we humans become more aware of the need to protect the delicate environmental balance of our planet, we are also learning that we ourselves are an environment, and have to protect our inner environment too.

The bacteria in our gut affect all aspects of our health, and they need to be guarded with great care for they are the very core not only of our immune system but our wellbeing.

There is a newly emerging understanding of the gut–lung axis, which links the state of the gut microbiome with health outcomes for the respiratory tract, and this relates to conditions such as cystic fibrosis and the inflammation of the lungs in Covid.[2] Both the gut and lungs share the same type of tissues, and amazingly, it has been found that when the microbiota of the gut is disturbed during an infection, the immune response in the lungs is also disturbed.

On the other hand, probiotic therapy has been found to significantly improve the outcome of lung diseases.[3] As such, certain probiotics reduce the viral load (number of viruses) in the body, enhance the immune response and calm down the deadly inflammatory response. Studies show that the Covid virus was directly subdued by common and easily available probiotics such as *Lactobacillus acidophilus*, *Bifidobacterium* and *Saccharomyces boulardii* which are found in foods such as live yoghurt, kimchi, and unpasteurized honey.[4]

There must be thousands, maybe millions of different bacterial species living harmoniously within our gut and all over our body, contributing towards the homeostasis of our body like a big friendly commune. So, when I prescribe probiotics for my patients, I like to use as wide a variety of bacterial species as possible because these friendly bacteria all contribute differently to our health, and I like to give the body as broad a chance as possible of recovery. The seeding of probiotics and the nourishing diet which I have discussed throughout this book make an excellent starting point to recovering your health. You can think of it like digging compost and manure into depleted soil. You restore the soil so that you can grow a beautiful garden full of strong plants, and healthy foods.

Anti-viral herbs

Garlic (*Allium sativum*)

Garlic is one of the most easily available natural anti-viral herbs that you can access. Its pungency is quite clearly inhospitable to invaders, making it effective against an impressive list of viruses, including adenovirus, influenza virus, coronavirus, herpes simplex virus and cytomegalovirus. In the olden days, it was even used to keep the witches away. Garlic prevents the virus entering into the cell. If the virus is already in the cell, then it restrains the virus from hijacking our RNA for reproduction, whilst at the same time, stimulating the immune system to attack and kill the invader.[5]

Garlic is well known to thin the blood, and may be useful for the micro-clotting which can still be relevant in Long Covid, especially if there is a hidden reservoir of viruses still causing trouble.

Garlic is one of my favourite foods when I catch a virus. This is what I do:

Toast a slice of rye bread.

Rub both sides thickly with raw garlic or, one side with a clove of crushed garlic.

Thinly slice a tomato and arrange on top of the toast.

Then drizzle with olive oil and crushed Himalayan salt.

Olive leaf (*Olea europaea*)

Olive leaves are cheap to come by, and if you happen to go on holiday to the Mediterranean, then I urge you to collect (with permission from the owner of the tree) a few handful of the leaves to dry and bring back against the cold and flu viruses.

A recent clinical trial measured the benefits of olive leaf extract on hospitalized Covid patients and found that olive leaf extract effectively reduced the fever, decreased the deadly inflammation whilst increasing blood oxygen levels, and thereby led to the early discharge of the patients. The olive leaf blocked the virus from entering the cells, and very importantly, it suppressed the massive inflammation that killed so many people with acute Covid.[6]

Olive leaf is used in cardiac disease to protect the blood vessels against inflammation and damage, thus in the case of a persistent virus which may be causing damage to the blood vessels, olive leaf tea is a excellent option for both preventing the virus from replicating, as well as helping to heal damaged blood vessels, and if you suffer from high blood pressure, then this really is the herb for you.

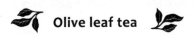

Olive leaf tea

Add half a teaspoon of dried leaf in a cup of boiling water.

Allow it to steep for 15 minutes, then strain and drink.

Add a few slices of fresh ginger and a little raw honey.

Do this twice a day to thwart viruses and support your heart

Lemon balm (*Melissa officinalis*)

This is a herb that I absolutely love to use, and I used it a lot when I helped people to recover from Covid. It has anti-viral properties, but it is also calming, and is so easy to grow in your own garden or even a pot on your windowsill.

For such a gentle little plant, it is a powerful destroyer of viruses, ably disarming HIV virus, herpes simplex virus, Epstein–Barr virus, and the SARS Covid virus by binding to the spike protein and blocking its entry and, therefore, its replication.[7] Lemon balm is also a powerful antioxidant, helping to bring down the inflammation caused by the viral infection.

Melissa has a marked calming effect on the nervous system, and bearing in mind that stress perpetuates fatigue and the vulnerability to severe viral infection, this makes lemon balm an excellent option to support your health with both Long Covid, and post-viral fatigue.

You can simply take lemon balm as a lovely afternoon tea, and also a bedtime tea to help you sleep. Any time that you feel stressed, enjoy another cup of lemon balm tea.

To make lemon balm tea, snip a sprig of the herb and drop it into a tea pot and cover so that the precious volatile oils don't waft away but are captured in your brew, because those volatile oils are where the action is with regards the anti-viral effect.

Elderberry (*Sambucus nigra*)

Elderberries are an absolute superfood when it comes to Covid and Long Covid. The berries are both anti-viral and packed with vitamin C. Elderberries not only prevent the invasion of the cell by the virus, but they rally the anti-viral arm of the immune system to rise up against the virus, and crucially, it is done without stimulating the deadly inflammatory cytokine storm.[8] This is very important because during an acute viral attack such as Covid, the inflammatory cytokine storm can be a killer.

For this reason, we don't want to use immune stimulants but rather immune modulators, preferably with powerful anti-viral properties, and even better, with blood vessel protective actions so as to prevent the blood from becoming sludgy and causing huge damage to the organs. The blue/ black anthocyanin pigment in the berry is of huge importance, because it protects and heals the lining of the blood vessels, which can become so dangerously damaged during a Covid infection.[9] In this way, elderberry helps to halt the infection, which also protects against the micro-clotting and massive tissue damage that ensues as a result.

Nature is absolutely marvellous by providing for all of this, for free and in abundance, at the end of the summer on our beloved elder trees.

When I am treating post-viral fatigue, I often use elderberries to treat the ongoing viral infection, and people get better. You can make an elderberry elixir to keep your family healthy. It is a very ancient recipe, absolutely delicious and tastes like mulled port.

 Elderberry Rob

Brewing Elderberry Rob is a wonderful way to spend an evening – filling your home with the juicy aroma of dark berries and spices.

In late summer, wander down the hedgerows and collect a basketful of ripe black elderberries. Back in the kitchen, pull the berries off the stalks with a fork, and fill a saucepan with your berries because you want a rich syrup. Just cover the top of the berries with water and gently simmer until they soften. Then crush the berries with a potato masher, or whizz them with a hand blender. Switch off the heat. Once cooled, strain off the berries pulp, but keep the dark purple liquid. Now reheat, and stir in as much sugar as you can until it will no longer dissolve. This is your preservative. Then, add a good amount of cinnamon, crushed cloves, quite a lot of fresh ginger, and a few star anise pods, and a few slices of lemon. Cover the pot, switch off the

heat and leave overnight to cool, then strain off the
spices and bottle the liquid.
    This delicious elixir can be taken every night over
winter as an anti-viral hot toddy. Because it is so
sweet, it is best mixed with a mug of boiling water,
using about 2 tablespoons of the Rob.

Turkey tail mushroom (*Trametes/Coriolus versicolor*)

It's a funny thing, but I notice that nature provides in abundance the exact herb that we will be needing later in the year. In recent years, I noticed a huge abundance of turkey tail mushrooms growing all over the forests, even on my garden furniture and the wooden boards of my herb beds. What a gift this herb is to those with both acute and Long Covid, and with ongoing fatigue as a result of Epstein–Barr virus or any other virus.

This interesting little mushroom, which looks like the fanned-out tail of a turkey (hence its common name), is a very clever medicine. It has anti-viral actions against a wide range of viruses such as HIV, Epstein–Barr virus (glandular fever), human papilloma virus, the herpes viruses, as well as being an immune modulator by stimulating the anti-viral aspects of our complex immune system, but down-regulating the inflammatory responses, and at the same time acting as an antioxidant.

The immune modulation prevents that immune over-reaction and the consequent massive inflammation which killed so many people during the Covid pandemic and many more during the Spanish Flu epidemic in 1918. This mushroom actually blocks the pro-inflammatory molecules in the body, and is so effective that it has found use in inflammatory bowel disease, osteoarthritis and traumatic brain injury[10].

Considering that with post-viral fatigue there may be a reservoir of lingering viruses which perpetuate the disease, and also neuro-inflammation, this herb is a very valuable asset to the recovery programme.

Shitake mushroom (*Lentinula edodes*)

The shitake mushroom is a medical mushroom that is delicious enough to be enjoyed as a culinary mushroom (as opposed to turkey tail which is definitely not a culinary mushroom). Medically, this mushroom can help us hugely during attack from a wide range of viruses, and has been shown to both enhance our immune response against the Covid virus whilst at the same time reducing inflammation in the lungs.[11]

Including even ordinary kitchen mushrooms in your diet can be very beneficial for those with post-viral brain fog, because all mushrooms, even white button mushrooms, protect and improve brain function and cognition.[12] This is very valuable because people with post-viral fatigue frequently struggle with brain fog and mental fatigue.

Wild mushrooms have a vast root-like mycelial web under the earth connecting plant root to plant root, like a huge communicating internet system, which is commonly referred to as the Wood-Wide-Web. The neurons in our brain look similar to trees with roots, and I find it fascinating that mushrooms connect our neurons just like they connect trees. Just as they facilitate the communication between the trees of a forest, so they do with the neurons of our brain.

Liquorice (*Glycyrrhiza glabra*)

Liquorice is one of my favourite herbs when treating post-viral fatigue, especially when there is adrenal fatigue. This lovely naturally sweet herb nourishes exhausted adrenal glands to help them to recover from their excessive output of cortisol.

At the same time, liquorice weakens and reduces the populations of a wide range of viruses and common yeasts such as Candida which are such a burden to one's health.[13]

Do bear in mind that if you have a high blood pressure, this herb is best avoided because it can increase blood pressure.

However, if you are one of those many people with chronic fatigue who feel dizzy especially when standing up, then liquorice can be extremely useful for you. In such cases there is usually low blood pressure or the inability for the body to compensate the blood flow when you stand up. I find that a pinch of Himalayan salt in a strong liquorice tea once or twice a day makes an enormous difference to those people.

The above herbs are just a small sample of some of the anti-viral herbs available, but these are very safe to use, effective and inexpensive.

Micro-clotting

The medical profession is trying hard to discover why people are suffering from Long Covid, and they think that it may be the result of a hidden reservoir of viruses which create tiny blood clots. The spike protein of the virus inflames and damages the lining of the blood vessels (the endothelium), which leads to bleeding and abnormal clotting activity. The micro-clots turn the blood into a thick sludge, which clogs up the capillaries, inhibiting the normal oxygen delivery to the tissues of the body. As a result there is shortness of breath, organ damage, brain fog and debilitating fatigue. These abnormal micro-clots can continue for months or even years after the initial infection.

Naturally, people are doing lots of research on the web from their homes, and have discovered that proteolytic (protein-dissolving) enzymes such as serrapeptase or nattokinase can dissolve clots. These are very safe natural medicines, far safer than over the counter aspirin, but unfortunately the EU and the UK have just decided to ban them. You can't help wondering sometimes.

Fortunately, food has not yet been banned, and there are proteolytic enzymes in pineapple and papaya which also dissolve clots. Bromelain is an enzyme found in raw pineapple stem and juice. Scientists found that it inhibits the Covid viral infection as well as dissolves blood clots.[14] Papaya also has an enzyme called papain which dissolves micro-clots, but it seems less effective than bromelain.[15]

Take care if you have an active gastric ulcer as the enzymes might exacerbate it. If you are on blood thinners, it would be best to ask your doctor if it is safe to eat pineapple because of the blood-thinning effects of both. But if you are free from both of the above problems, then you can either eat raw pineapple, kiwi and papaya or make smoothies from the fruits. The key is to eat these fruits on an empty stomach because if there is milk or any other protein in your stomach, the enzyme will break this down instead of the micro-clots. The same goes for the smoothie – just whizz the fruits in water, not milk because milks have proteins. See a recipe below.

Healing damaged blood vessels

Anthocyanins are natural compounds commonly found in food, and in particular the dark berries such as elderberries, blackberries, blueberries, mulberries, blackcurrants, raspberries and strawberries. Anthocyanins are antioxidant and therefore anti-inflammatory, and in particular, they protect and heal the inner lining of the endothelium.

One study showed that by combining bromelain and anthocyanins, the damage to the endothelium was alleviated, resulting in better oxygenation of the tissues.[16] Another study found that the anthocyanins in berries such as strawberry and raspberry were able to block and inhibit the virus entry and activity.[17]

Blackberries are abundantly available at the end of summer and they are bursting with anthocyanins. Do go out and collect bags of the berries. You can freeze them and use a handful every day in a juice, as I am about to describe below, to heal and strengthen your blood vessels.

Pineapple, papaya and berry smoothie

3 thick slices of fresh pineapple
½ a papaya or a kiwi fruit
A handful of the dark berries of your choice

*Add your fruits to the blender and then enough
water to be able to reduce this to a slush. With this
smoothie, you have the added bonus of the fruit
fibre, which feeds your friendly gut bacteria in your
colon. A double whammy of goodness!*

*Remember to take this smoothie on an empty
stomach, and the easiest time is about an hour
before breakfast. It is also very important that the
juice is freshly pressed because enzymes do have a
shelf life, so make it and drink it.*

Hawthorn (*Crategus spp*)

The Covid virus is well known to attack the heart, and
therefore it makes absolute sense to use a herb which is
famously beneficial to the heart, and rich in anthocyanins.

A study, investigating the effects of various medical
herbs on the symptoms of Long Covid, demonstrated how
hawthorn berries reduce palpitations and breathlessness
whilst improving tolerance of exercise.[18] Another study
on hawthorn confirms that it strengthens the integrity
and function of the endothelium, inhibiting endothelial
inflammation and reducing blood clotting,[19] which are exactly
the effects required for healing.

I have used hawthorn berries for people struggling with
cardiac symptoms following a Covid infection and those
people have shown very significant improvements. Hawthorn
berries are safe, and easy to find at the end of summer. They
can be collected, dried and made into a herbal tea.

Hawthorn, elderberry and rosehip tea

This is a brilliant tea which will improve your immune system, fight the lurking viruses, and heal your blood vessel walls.

Collect a basket of hawthorn, elderberries and rosehips in the late summer and dry these in the airing cupboard, over your Aga, or somewhere dry and warm. If you prefer, rinse them, dry them thoroughly and then keep them in the freezer.

Every day you can simply drop ½ tsp of elder-berries, 5 hawthorn berries, and a few rosehips into a cup of boiling water, leave for 20 minutes and strain and enjoy. Add a little blueberry cordial if you want to improve the taste.

Turmeric (*Curcuma longa*)

I love to watch how herbs are used by the indigenous people of the land, because they know exactly what to do with them. In India, the mama's use turmeric powder, with black pepper and ghee or coconut oil to make their medicines, and guess what – that is exactly what we need to absorb the turmeric, and to heal our bodies.

Turmeric contains a constituent called curcumin which has been much studied for its anti-cancer, anti-inflammatory actions. It is also anti-viral, and restores the correct balance of the immune system.[20] So turmeric splendidly ticks all the boxes that we need for recovery from Covid, but there is a big problem. Curcumin is very poorly absorbed because liver enzymes break down the curcumin before it can be absorbed. However, there are two tricks which will enormously improve the adsorption of curcumin by the body.

Piperine, a constituent of black pepper, blocks that liver enzyme breakdown, allowing curcumin to be far better absorbed. Even a tiny amount like ¼ of a teaspoon, or even a pinch, increases curcumin absorption by 2,000%.

Herbalists like to use whole plant extracts. By this we mean that nothing is taken out or added to the product. We believe that all the hundreds or thousands of plant constituents work together synergistically to produce perfect medicine, and there is a saying which goes, "The whole is more than the sum of its parts." But many companies say that it is curcumin alone which does all the good work, and so they isolate it from the rest of the turmeric root, selling it at a rather high price.

However, the fresh root, and even turmeric powder contains turmeric oils, which improve the bio availability of curcumin by seven times. If you take turmeric with black pepper and fat, the breakdown of the molecule is blocked and curcumin is far better absorbed.

One thing to consider is that curcumin stays in the bloodstream for approximately three hours, so to maintain the benefits, you would need to take it about five times a day.

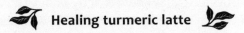 **Healing turmeric latte**

1 tsp of fresh turmeric root grated, or ½ tsp
    turmeric powder
A good grind of black pepper
1 tsp of ghee or coconut butter
(I like to add extra spices like star anise, cinnamon
    and/or nutmeg, all of which have therapeutic
    properties)

Melt the fat in the small saucepan. Add the pepper, turmeric and other spices. Gently warm the spices, mixing them into the melted fat until you can smell the spices.

Now add a cup of coconut milk and warm, allowing the turmeric to turn the milk a beautiful

sunshine yellow. Turn off the heat and allow the
extraction to continue for a few minutes. Add a
little raw honey if you wish, then strain and enjoy.

I have used scientific studies to prove to you that all the herbs and foods listed above will be very helpful for your home healing of post-viral fatigue, especially Long Covid. Do make sure that you include these healing herbs and foods into your diet as they are safe and effective. Please do not under estimate how healing these foods can be. Considering there really isn't a medicine out there to help people to recover from Long Covid, these healing plants offer an excellent option, and they are safe and nourishing.

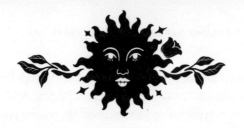

CHAPTER 11

HEALING THE BRAIN

It wasn't very long ago when chronic fatigue was thought of as being "all in the mind" – and it turns out that it is! Or at least a significant aspect of fatigue is generated in the brain. It is now recognized that much of the fatigue is driven by an inflamed brain, and certain inflammatory molecules show a connection with fatigue and depression.[1]

Gut–brain axis

The "gut–brain axis" refers to a two-way flow of communication between the two body systems. Our gut sends a message of emptiness to the brain, which instructs us to find food, and of course, we have all experienced the loosening of the bowels associated with anxiety generated in the brain. So the two-way communication along the nerve route is clear, but what is not so well known is that the flora and fauna in our gut communicate with our brain too, and send messages to the brain concerning sleep, memory, mood and much more.

An imbalanced gut environment with too many unhealthy bacteria (dysbiosis) can result in depression and fatigue.[2] Dysbiosis triggers inflammation in the gut, leading to increased permeability, and this allows toxins from the unfriendly bacteria to leak into the bloodstream and across the blood-brain barrier into the brain, triggering neuro-inflammation. The result is fatigue, sadness, anxiety and loss of motivation.[3]

However, the brilliant news is that scientists have discovered a new type of brain nerve cell which actually protects the brain against inflammation when it receives information from friendly bacteria in the healthy gut.[4]

Consider starting with *Saccharomyces boulardii*: a friendly yeast which sweeps out the unfriendly bacteria and yeasts. Then, very elegantly, this yeast itself dies, having left a cleaner gut ready to be seeded with billions of friendly bacteria. After the *Saccharomyces boulardii*, take a wide range of good-quality probiotics, and I would suggest continuing this for two to six months, at least.

Food for the brain

A great way of bringing these very helpful bacteria into your gut is by eating them. Foods such as sauerkraut, or drinking kefir, kombucha, natto, kvass, apple cider vinegar, tempeh, miso, kimchi or live yoghurts all provide a wide variety of friendly bacteria, and a wide range is healthy for us.

Alongside your probiotic regime, remember to follow the highly antioxidant Rainbow Diet, including lots of lovely colourful fruits and vegetables. The vegetable fibres act as prebiotics, providing food for the probiotics.

Please make stringent efforts to avoid sugar and junk food, which only feeds unfriendly gut microbes, fuels inflammation and perpetuates your illness. Remember to keep your blood sugar levels even by eating good-quality food, little and often, so that you never find yourself in the situation of craving sugary foods for an energy boost.

Omega-3

Essential fatty acids are specific fats derived from foods, which are essential for our health, but our bodies are unable to manufacture them. The omega-3 fatty acids are a class of essential fatty acids which have many benefits for our body. But before I break them down, I just want to point out four major benefits of omega-3 fatty acids, with regards everything that you have been reading so far.

1. They are integral components of the phospholipid bilayer which forms the membrane surrounding our mitochondria and cell walls, and therefore protects your energy.

2. They have healthy anti-clotting actions, so that the blood cells slip past each other instead of clumping together into blood clots.

3. They help to heal the lining of your blood vessels as well as making the blood cells healthy again.

4. The omega-3 essential fatty acids can reduce neuro-inflammation and nourish the brain tissues, in that way inhibiting cognitive decline whilst positively influencing the mood.[5]

Omega-3 oils are made up of 3 components:

Eicosapentaenoic acid (EPA) – exerts an anti-inflammatory effect in our bodies and helps to rebalance the disrupted immune system. It is very important in restricting the neuro-inflammation in the brain and inflammation throughout the body.

Docosahexaenoic acid (DHA) – is very important to support brain function, as well as calming the neuro-inflammation in the brain. It helps to heal the blood vessel walls and halt micro-clotting, so you can see that it could be absolutely lifesaving. DHA exerts an anti-inflammatory effect on the body, and reduces post-exercise muscle soreness, and as anyone with chronic fatigue knows, muscle pain is very much a part of the picture.

Foods rich in DHA and EPA include herring, sardines, tuna, salmon, trout, krill oil and algae oil.

Alpha-linolenic acid (ALA) – can be converted into EPA and DHA, but it only converts into tiny amounts in our bodies. ALA is found in kale, walnuts, hemp and chia seeds, and soya beans.

I like to use food as medicine, but in this case, I think that supplements with very good-quality fish oils or algae oil are necessary to achieve the therapeutic effect needed to exert a healing effect on the body, and to turn these horrible illnesses around.

This is very important. When purchasing omega-3 oils, don't be tempted by a cheap product. Rather buy the best you can afford, because the seas are filled with pollutants these days. The liver of the fish is very rich in oils, but of course that is where the toxins are broken down by the body. I like to buy my fish oils produced from Nordic countries where the seas are clean, and they have been purified using gentle methods. Some of the cheaper oils may have higher levels of toxins, which only adds to your toxic burden. So if you buy cheap fish oils, you could be buying concentrated sea toxins. Rather take a lower dose of expensive oils if you need to spread the cost, and try to eat wild oily fish such as sardines, mackerel, herrings, trout, or sardines and tuna, which are not too expensive. If you prefer a plant-based diet, then include freshly ground flaxseeds, chia seeds, walnuts and algae oil in your recovery programme.

Vitamin B complex

There are eight B vitamins, each of which have important and different functions in our body and are of particular importance to our nervous system. These vitamins are well known for reducing the feelings of stress and anxiety, whilst nourishing a depleted nervous system. Stress itself burns up the B vitamins, and if you are low in B vitamins then a supplement can help to alleviate brain fog, memory and fatigue

Coconut oil

Coconut oil is rich in medium chain fatty acids, which are broken down to form ketones. When the body is struggling to provide energy from glucose, it can use an alternative source of energy in the form of ketones.[6] So coconut oil can provide the brain with this alternative energy source if it is deficient in glucose, and it seems that in both Long Covid and chronic fatigue syndrome sufferers, some (but not all) people have altered glucose metabolism.

However, coconut oil has more to offer. It is also high in antioxidants, and has been shown to reduce CRP levels (an inflammatory marker commonly used by doctors).[7] It also has anti-fungal, anti-bacterial effects, and blocks the reproduction of viruses, specifically Covid virus.[8] [9]

Chocolate

In ancient Mexico, the chocolate tree was planted by a great feathered serpent god as a divine gift for the Aztec and Toltec people. The Aztec ruler, Montezuma II, famously drank many cups a day from his golden goblet, and it was referred to as "the divine drink which builds resistance and fights fatigue". They said of it that a man can walk all day without food if he drank chocolate. Later when it was brought back to Europe, Carl Linnaeus named it Theobroma cacao (Theo = God and Broma = food), therefore naming chocolate as "food of the Gods".

Chocolate has many benefits for our wellbeing as most people happily acknowledge. Cocoa holds a gentle stimulant called theobromine, which dilates the blood vessels, increasing blood flow to the brain. By increasing the blood flow to the brain, with the subsequent increase of oxygen and extra nutrition delivery to the brain cells, we experience improved cognition and neuroplasticity.[10] Neuroplasticity can be thought of as the re-wiring of the brain. It refers to the ability of the brain to reorganize itself and adapt to new circumstances or to change the way it responds to stimuli such as anxiety triggers.

The extra nutrition delivered to the brain cells enhances brain function. The improved blood flow also delivers the other amazing natural chemicals found in chocolate such as a rich range of antioxidants; in fact, chocolate has higher levels of antioxidants than blueberries or green tea, and thus helps to reduce the inflammation in the brain.

Another constituent of chocolate is phenylethylamine (PEA) which increases sensations of pleasure and reward. PEA is referred to as the "love molecule" because it increases that glorious feeling of being in love.

Chocolate increases the delivery of serotonin, which sends signals between our brain nerve cells helping to stabilize our mood so that we feel calmer and happier, and more able to focus.

Another chocolate chemical is anandamide, commonly referred to as the "bliss chemical", because it banishes anxiety and reduces pain sensations. It almost takes us to a heavenly place in our minds. Black pepper contains the alkaloid guineesine, which blocks the breakdown of anandamide, thereby increasing or prolonging its blissful effects. More about this bliss chemical later.

Studies on young people and chronic fatigue sufferers showed that chocolate improved mental performance and reduced fatigue symptoms in chronic fatigue syndrome.[11] [12]

Of course, ordinary high-sugar milk chocolate is not going to have these benefits. Ideally, you should drink unroasted cacao, or eat raw chocolate with a low sugar content.

Brain restoratives herbs

Lion's mane mushroom

Lion's mane is a splendid-looking fungi, which looks nothing like a mushroom, but rather like an elegant frozen waterfall. What is fascinating is that when you cut this mushroom in half, it looks like a brain, as do several herbs which are used to help with cognition.

As a medicine, it is a very valuable, because it reduces inflammation in the brain, and heals the nerves as well as promoting nerve regrowth. The result is significant improvement in focus, concentration and memory, markedly improving cognition.[13] [14] [15]

One study showed how a group of menopausal women had lowered levels of depression and anxiety after eating lion's mane cookies for four weeks.[16] What an excellent idea to integrate the lion's mane into your daily diet. I make this hot chocolate for myself when I feel tired, and it helps with mental fatigue.

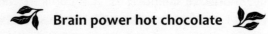

Brain power hot chocolate

2 capsules (1/3 tsp) of lion's mane powder
A pinch of chilli powder
1 heaped tsp of raw cacao powder
1/3 tsp of coconut oil
Xylitol, stevia or honey to taste
1 cup of boiling water
A splash of milk or cream (dairy or vegan)

Put all the ingredients into the cup and give it a
good whisk, and enjoy.

Lemon balm (*Melissa officinalis*)

We are now familiar with this lovely plant which has always been a kind friend to the jittery exhausted person. In previous chapters, we have considered how this herb is an effective anti-viral, a calming herb, and now we see that it can also improve cognitive function, and decrease neuro-inflammation.[17] [18] However, it seems to work even more effective for brain function when combined with rosemary. The scientists made special note of the antioxidant ability of the herb to calm the neuro-inflammation and degeneration of brain tissue associated with the aging brain, but we can extrapolate that to the loss of cognition due to the neuro-inflammation of post-viral or adrenal fatigue.

It is a very safe herb and one that you can use with confidence. The only time I would urge care is if you have a low thyroid function because *Melissa* can block the thyroid hormones.

Rosemary (*Rosmarinus officinalis*)

Shakespeare said it when he wrote, "There's rosemary, that's for remembrance". It has ever been thus. Since ancient Egypt, the herb has been used in funeral ceremonies to preserve and remember the deceased, and the ancient Greek students would circle garlands of it upon their heads to facilitate their memories. Stroke the plant, and the tangy aroma will immediately lift your spirits.

Long associated with memory, rosemary is a powerful antioxidant, helping to alleviate the neuro-inflammation, especially when associated with Long Covid because it is also able to inhibit blood clotting.

Rosemary improves circulation to the brain, and in doing so, delivers oxygen,[19] which results in enhanced cognition, alertness and mood. Taking rosemary can be as simple as taking a herbal tea, or sniffing the essential oil.

Very similarly to sage, it defends against Alzheimer's disease and possibly Parkinson's disease, by protecting the neurons and restraining amyloid plaque formation.

For younger people, vaporized rosemary essential oil significantly improves short-term memory, feeling mentally fresher, more alert.[20] Rosemary changes our brainwaves from the quiet and restful alpha state to the problem-solving beta waves, where we are attentive and focused.

An interesting study compared the effects of rosemary with peppermint and lavender essential oils. In accordance with tradition, the rosemary and peppermint improved short-term memory of the group, whilst the lavender worsened it, but made everyone feel calm and relaxed.[21] However, to be focused, you need to feel calm. I love to combine all three to bring a refreshing calming atmosphere into my workspace. You can do this for yourself by either using a vaporizer or just adding a few drops to a tissue.

CAUTION: Rosemary should not be used in any way if you have epilepsy, as it may trigger a seizure.

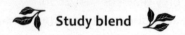 **Study blend**

4 drops rosemary essential oil
3 drops lavender essential oil
2 drops peppermint (or lemon) essential oil

These essential oils can be added to a diffuser so that they gently fill the air with their beautiful fragrance and benefits. If you don't have a diffuser, just drops onto a tissue and place on your desk.

Lavender (*Lavendula angustifolia*)

Lavender has the opposite effect to the rosemary, where it seems to slow the reaction time and calm the red-alertness of the brain (20), however, this is a very useful effect. People who have been stressed for a long time, even burnt out with normal everyday racing-around type of stress, are too speedy. Their brains have forgotten how to slow down, and they feel over-stimulated and frazzled. In these cases, lavender is a blessing (actually, all herbs are a blessing), because it gives you a brain-break. It brings the peacefulness and quiet so craved by the wired and tired brain.

Lavender essential oil is easy to use. Just drop a dot on your collar, or on a tissue near to where you are working or resting. You can add some to your bath water by mixing a few drops with Epsom salts to help to calm your brain waves.

St John's wort (*Hypericum perfoliatum*)

Once upon a time when I studied herbal medicine, the college was in an old mansion deep in the countryside, far away from anywhere. In that house lived a little old man and a little old woman, and they taught us herbal medicine. Mr Zeylstra didn't only teach us that St John's wort was an anti-depressant, he taught us that it is a nervous system tropho-restorative. That means that it restores the nervous system.

When you have been so stressed for so long that your nervous system feels stripped out and raw, like electric wires without the insulation covering, then St John's wort soothes and heals the nerves. Of course, when your nervous system is so debilitated, you are bound to feel low in mood, because you can barely function. But depression in this case is not the underlying problem. You are depressed because you are ill, not the other way around. So many of my patients these days feel that way, I am afraid. But herbs change that.

With Long Covid and post-viral fatigue there are viruses which may have penetrated even into the brain tissues, causing inflammation and nerve damage. St John's wort has the added bonus of being an excellent anti-viral herb, alleviating inflammation and healing nerve tissue, as well as helping to restore the natural brain chemistry.[22]

Ginger (*Zingiber officinalis*)

During the Covid pandemic, ginger doubled in price. In those days, if you saw fresh ginger, you pounced on it and bought it straight away because everybody was buying ginger and turmeric. Of course, when the media did not stop telling you that there was a deadly virus everywhere, which had a high chance of killing you and your family, but doctors and pharmacies told you to go home and take paracetamol – guess what? You are going to hop onto the internet and look at other options. Ginger and turmeric were available, not too expensive and seemed to offer some benefits.

Ginger has direct, powerful, anti-viral actions and is able to power up the immune system against the virus, making this kitchen herb very useful when you have a lingering community of viruses perpetuating your illness. Indeed, a study in China showed that patients who were given 1.5g of ginger twice a day but had the same treatment as others, left hospital after a significantly shorter period than other patients.[23]

Ginger has many benefits, including that it is antioxidant and anti-inflammatory and has been shown in other illnesses, such as Alzheimers, multiple sclerosis and Parkinson's disease, to protect the central nervous system from the damaging effects of such diseases.[24]

Turmeric (*Curcuma longa*)

A study in Brazil found that 10g of turmeric increased oxygenation of the brain by 42%, and blood flow by a whopping

54%.[25] Bearing in mind that the damaged blood vessel walls result in micro-clotting of the blood, which means that the sludgy blood is unable to delivery oxygen and nutrients to the brain. As a result, those cells will suffer significant injury, which no doubt accounts for some of the mental symptoms such as brain fatigue, difficulty finding words, and struggling to think clearly.

Sage (*Salvia officinalis*)

Sage is not called that for nothing. It has long been used to enhance cognition in the aging brain. One of the ways it helps is by inhibiting the accumulation of the amyloid-β peptide, which is so significant in the development of Alzheimer's disease. However, for our purposes, it is also one of those antioxidant and circulatory stimulant herbs which support brain function.[26]

Sage, and nettle seeds too for that matter, help to prevent the breakdown of an important neurotransmitter called acetylcholine. In doing so, they contribute towards the preservation of memory, attention, learning and motivation. In other words, these herbs help to keep you "bright". This interesting study showed how a low dose of one 300mg capsule of sage reduced anxiety whilst the higher dose of two 300mg capsules brought about an enhancement of alertness, calmness and contentedness.[27]

Elegantly, sage also happens to be an anti-viral herb, and rather famously helps with menopausal symptoms, which can also be associated with the distressing symptoms of memory loss and brain fog.

Nettle seeds (*Urtica dioica*)

Within those little green clusters of seeds lie a superfood waiting to provide you with lusty vigour. The seeds hold omega-3, -6 and -9 fatty acids, giving not only the brain, but the cardiac system a nice boost of omegas.

We all know that nettles contain histamine – the chemical that is responsible for the sting, and you will probably not be surprised to note that histamine acts as an excitatory chemical, stimulating arousal in the brain and the whole body.

Now this is interesting, because there goes a story about a doctor in charge of an old-age care home who insisted that the nurses put one teaspoon of nettle seeds on the residents' morning porridge. Apparently, they became "lusty". It is not elaborated whether this was in song or inclination, but the nettle seeds certainly perked up their petals.

This is why herbalists use nettle seeds. It is specifically indicated for those who feel mentally tired, jaded and worn out. The seeds are particularly used for those who experience "brain fatigue".

Whilst nettles are the enemy of gardeners, medical herbalists love this herb, and it is one of my favourite herbs to collect, because somehow it imparts to me that feeling of "being in flow". The lovely green fragrance soothes my mind, and even the occasional sting is not taken with offence by my exposed skin.

In the springtime, we use the young leaves because they provide a good boost of minerals and vitamins, as well as acting as a blood cleanser, which is what we need after stodgy winter food. But in the winter months, we need nourishment of a different kind. We need healthy fats and a tonic to get us through the long, dark, cold days, and so the nettle seeds can be included in your food. I find the easiest way to include nettle seeds is to put them into my salt grinder, and little by little they soak into my body.

The poet Thomas Campbell (1777–1884) wrote: "In Scotland, I have eaten nettles, I have slept in nettle sheets, and I have dined off a nettle tablecloth. The young and tender nettle is an excellent potherb. The stalks of the old nettle are as good as flax for making cloth. I have heard my mother say that she thought nettle cloth more durable than any other species of linen."

The underlying cause is key: after examining why people with chronic fatigue and Long Covid develop neuro-inflammation, a group of scientists concluded that: "All these responses relate to how each individual's immune system reacts to the external stressor – and that is the common factor in the development of the illnesses."[28]

That stressor which disrupts the immune system and makes people so ill for so long is not necessarily a mental or emotional stress. The stress is something that keeps us under constant strain, such as an ongoing low-grade viral infection, mould toxins in the house, or heavy metal poisoning, being over-worried about exams, or grief over the loss of a loved one. The stress could be that unrecognized type that the modern person doesn't even realize, and that is when we keep going, ignoring our body's cry to stop and rest, until one day a virus strikes and we simply cannot get out of bed that day, nor the next, nor for many months or even years to come.

This is the hardest thing that I will have to say in this book, but the underlying stressor in your life may be people close to you. I am very sorry to say this, but sometimes relationships become toxic and very draining, and then you have to find a way to create a distance from that person or persons, because they are making you very ill. It is also possible that you are their stressor. Sometimes one is able to talk to them calmly, go to counselling together, or draw some clear boundaries, but I have known some of my patients who have had to cut off ties, or create very distant ties with short telephone conversations at best. One dear person even ran away and hid at a friend's home in another county, because her relationship with her sister was making her so ill.

Hopefully, with time, these relationships can be healed, but sometimes we have to let them go with love. That is the key – not holding on to bitterness and hatred, but let them go with love, so that they can get on with their life and you with yours. Pierre Pradervand wrote a beautiful book titled, *The Gentle Art of Blessing* (Simon & Schuster, 2009), which discusses the healing benefits of blessing those who cause you pain.

Over the years, I have noticed over and over again that the immune system is not able to overcome the viral infection, etc., because it is already exhausted and disrupted, following a time of previous unremitting stress. So, please do pay attention to the restorative herbs that you can use, but above all – examine your life, try to find what it is that is causing your system to feel over-stressed and deal with that. Then you can start to heal yourself with these herbs from your kitchen and garden.

Other ways to calm and restore your brain

A study on the brain waves during sleep of people with chronic fatigue showed that their abnormal alpha and delta waves impaired brain wave homeostasis, resulting in unremitting fatigue, unrefreshing sleep, generalized pain, discomfort and impaired memory.[29]

This is a key bit of information, because several studies also show disturbed brain waves, and so we can conclude that restoring brain wave homeostasis will be a vital ingredient to the healing of the brain, particularly if mental or emotional stress, over work or over-conscientiousness are the underlying factors.

Remember that the brain (the central nervous system) is the great conductor of our body's functioning. Let's imagine that it is the conductor of a magnificent orchestra (that is you!). If the conductor is reeling with fatigue and confused brain waves, how can s/he possibly conduct the beautiful performance that s/he is tasked to do? The whole piece of music will be out of tune and jarring. As such, we must sooth and nourish our inner conductor, so that we can start to heal our brain and our lives.

Sound Therapy

Music is well known to affect our brain waves, and calming music has a significantly positive effect on restoring our brain waves, and in fact calms the brain much faster than silence.[30] Think about the tranquil peace of a monastery. You can bring that peace into your home with some incense and the healing music of Tibetan Buddhist chanting, or Gregorian chants.

Solfeggio frequencies are particular sound patterns which interact with your brain to bring about peace, focus and cellular healing. The frequencies themselves are not that interesting to listen to, but when embedded in gentle music, they really can have a very positive effect on our brain waves. These frequencies can easily be found on YouTube, and played via your phone to create a near instant effect on your brain. Using music, you can almost immediately transform the fizzing of over-stimulation to the respite of a calmer, more cohesive brain vibration.

If you find music too stimulating, you may prefer some ambient background sounds instead. This is a way of creating a serene soundscape around yourself which can cocoon you from the hectic noises of modern life. Perhaps play around with soundscapes such as Medieval Scriptorium, Cosy Winter Cabin with Log Fire, Monastery Garden, Whales in the Ocean, Desert Sands or whatever soundscape you feel appeals to you. Choose a soundscape which you feel will comfort your brain and allow it to float peacefully in a calm atmosphere.

Laughter

Laughter floods our systems with hormones of joy, which send messages to our brain that life is good and there is something to laugh about. Laughter changes our state of mind. Sometimes I think that we take life far too seriously, and even myself, I have found that, if I feel a bit grumpy or frustrated, if I make a silly joke at myself, my mood immediately changes for the better and my day is improved as a result. You may choose to laugh with people, just see the funny side of life, or watch comedians on YouTube. Whichever way you choose – try to laugh and lift your spirits. There is a saying that laughter is the best medicine. I think it is excellent medicine, but I think love is the very best medicine.

Share love

We don't have to be in love to share love with everyone and everything. I often think that when we raise our hand to wave at someone over the street, we are unconsciously sending them love, and then they send some back! That makes both of you feel good. When we are friendly to the lady at the post office or kind to our neighbour, or even send a blessing of kindness to someone whose company is not particularly enjoyable, it brings love into the world. A feeling of goodness warms like a candle flame in your heart, spreading that light and love out into the world.

Fill your world with the love and light from your own heart, and truly, you will make your world and the rest of the world a brighter place. Nothing heals like love. Love is the greatest power there is. Love and plants.

Forest bathing

Forest bathing is a beautiful way to spend a few hours. If you are lucky enough to live near a forest, you can simply walk amongst the trees until you feel called to a special spot. There you make yourself comfortable, especially if you can lean against a tree, and then allow your mind to rest in the energy of the trees. Remembering that they are much older than us, and much taller than us, so they have a long over-view of life. Maybe you would like to try to tune into a tree, or the forest and ask, "What is it all about?"

Even if you don't want to think – just enjoy the fragrance of the forest. Did you know that the smell of the forest is rich in volatile oils released by the trees called phytoncides? These chemicals are fabulous because when we breathe them in, they enhance our immune system, especially the anti-viral and anti-tumour side of the immune system. So forest bathing calms our mind, and rebalances our immune system.

White and green noise

If you can't get to a forest, it is always possible to open a window and listen to the birds. Who knows what they are chattering about, but focusing on their chirruping, squeaks and squeals delights the mind and gives you a brain-break. Even listening to the wind is a form of "green noise" therapy.

If you are unable to access the wind, the trees or the birds, "white and green sounds" can be found on YouTube, and these frequencies help to distract our attention from other disruptive and harsh noises such as traffic.

Whilst white sound has an equal intensity, giving it a constant "shhhh" sound, green noise is a deeper sound, more akin to the sounds of nature such as the wind in the leaves of a forest, or rain.

These sound frequencies have been studied for several decades because they have a calming effect on the central nervous system, helping people to sleep better and to focus in a calm, cohesive manner.

When people have chronic fatigue, they sometimes crave sensory deprivation, and outside noises can be a form of torture to the utterly exhausted brain. Allowing your brain to rest in white or green sound may be like taking your brain on retreat.

Earthing

Getting your fingers in the soil, growing something or taking care of plants is therapeutic because you are nurturing an undemanding other being. However, there is another significant benefit to getting your hands into the soil, and it is called "earthing".

I know that it may sound a bit woo-woo, but it is not. We are electrical beings. That is a fact. Our brain and heart are an electromagnetic system, as is our planet Earth. We should be perfectly attuned to the electromagnetic field of the Earth, except that now with all the electrical equipment around us, our electrical attunment is disrupted, and we feel very out of sorts. The problem is that we have grown up with this disruption and have got so used to feeling out of sorts electrically that we don't actually know how we ought to feel. It is only after spending time with our bare feet or hands on the Earth that our electromagnetic energies are realigned again with the Earth and we remember how good we feel when we are connect with the Earth.

The surface of the Earth is covered in a vast supply of electrons, from which our modern lifestyle has disconnected us, and some research is proving what most of us already know, which is that our disconnection from the Earth is a major contributor to the dysfunctioning and unwellness of our state of being.

Reconnecting with the Earth's abundance of negatively charged electrons enables those harmonious electrical rhythms to flow directly from the Earth into our bodies, and, can you believe it – they act as natural antioxidants, neutralizing the positively charged inflammatory free radicals. In doing so, earthing normalizes our daily cortisol rhythm, significantly improves sleep and reduces pain and inflammation. Earthing even affects our mineral levels, so that the mineral content in our blood, and even thyroid hormones, are raised after a single night of earthing.[31] [32] [33]

Go on retreat

Going on retreat is just that. You are retreating from your normal life, and reconnecting with something sacred within you. You may not choose to go on a spiritual retreat, but then again, you may feel that calling to spend time in a monastery or on a yoga or meditation retreat. Myself, I love to get into the African bush, and I go on safari whenever I can. I try to get as deep into the bush and as far away from civilization as I can, so that for a few days I am able to surrender my whole being into the embrace of Africa. There I fall into the rhythms of the sun rising and setting, the animals' response to that, the tangy scent of the herbage, and the distant (or not so distant) early morning roars of the lions. I attune to the buzzing of insects, the warmth of the sandy soil on the soles of my feet, and my eyes resting on far horizons. The last time I went, I was exhausted after a very busy period during the Covid years. I desperately needed a brain-break for an extended period of time, and I remember telling my partner that all I needed to think about was not being eaten, and what's for lunch. Safari feeds my soul like nothing else can, and I encourage you to visit that place which feeds your soul and gives your whole being a break.

Some people find this on the snowy slopes of high mountains. Others find it diving in the oceans, or walking on a pilgrimage. You might like to go on a writers' retreat, or learning a craft where you are using the creative aspect of your brain rather than the thinking side.

If you feel drawn to a retreat, but don't know much about them, try reading *The Good Retreat Guide* by Stafford Whiteaker (Hay House UK Ltd) which is an excellent reference book describing a wide variety of retreats. In fact, just browsing through the pages and fantasizing about which one you would love to go on, with a gentle cup of tea, is in itself a momentary retreat.

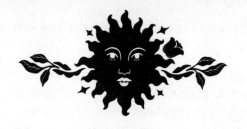

CHAPTER 12

STRESS, PAIN AND THE ENDOCANNABINOID SYSTEM

Unbelievably, the endocannabinoid system (ECS) was only discovered in 1988. A whole body system, hidden in plain sight. Your endocannabinoid system is a bit like the mafia. It's everywhere, but you can't see it, and yet it controls everything! This system is less about structure and more about action, then again, not even action, but rather balancing and tempering. It is not a collection of tissues, but fast acting molecules with receptors located on cells throughout your body: in the brain, the nerves, white blood cells, connective tissues and the glands. In fact, this system is so important that it has regulated the homeostatic balance of your brain throughout your life.[1]

One of the reasons why we hear so little about it, is because it was named after that controversial plant *Cannabis sativa*, from which the molecule tetrahydrocannabinol (THC) is derived. It was that molecule which led to the discovery of this wide-acting and mysterious system.

The use of cannabis goes back over 12,000 years to the nomadic peoples of the Altai Mountains in central Asia,[2] but in the last hundred years, the war on drugs transformed this esteemed plant into an illegal substance. Thus the body system named after cannabis became something of an embarrassment and was shushed up. Now, as the world reels with stress, pain, anxiety and fatigue, the plant is coming back into favour.

The endocannabinoid system is subtle and ethereal. You can't see it, but you can't do without it. It is the benign controller of our glandular, immune and nervous system, protecting us from the effects of stress, and conversely, too much stress suppresses our endocannabinoid tone. We all have an underlying endocannabinoid tone, but sometimes our tone becomes undermined, and this can profoundly affect our wellbeing. Not least, some disease conditions which up until now have had no known cause; many of which are very closely related to stress and chronic fatigue.

What is the endocannabinoid system?

The ECS is a complex system of molecular signals, produced by our body to stimulate a vast network of receptors. It is involved in the modulation of pain, inflammation, immune responses, cancer, mood disorders and intestinal motility. So far, two types of cannabinoid receptors have been discovered in the body.

1. CB1 receptors, which are richly distributed in the brain, spinal cord and on the mitochondria. In fact, in the brain, there are more CB1 receptors than any other type of receptor. They control the other neurotransmitter (signalling molecules) levels of activity.

2. CB2 receptors are found mainly in the immune system, along the gastro-intestinal tract, and nerves outside of the central nervous system; they are critical to helping balance our immune response, and play a role in calming bowel inflammation, contraction and pain.

The endocannabinoids

Whilst cannabis has a wide range of molecules called cannabinoids, our body produces its own molecules which are extremely similar, and are thus called endocannabinoids. Endo means "within", so these are cannabinoids made within our own body. Both cannabinoids and endocannabinoids are able to dock into the endocannabinoid receptors of our body, and influence our mood, pain and immune responses.

There are two main types of endocannabinoid molecules thus far identified, but about 160 types of phytocannabinoids (plant cannabinoids). You can ignore the number of phytocannabinoids discovered because the number keeps changing, but you can see that there are a lot of plant cannabinoids, and they are found mostly in cannabis, but also other plants like echinacea, chocolate and black pepper.

The first endocannabinoid discovered was named anandamide – the bliss chemical, after the Sanskrit word "ananda", meaning bliss. This word is important because it emphasizes that within your own body, you have the capacity to create your inner bliss.

The endocannabinoid system has several known actions, but the actions depend on where the receptor is located and which endocannabinoid binds to it. For example, endocannabinoids on the CB1 receptors in a spinal nerve will relieve pain, while others binding to a CB2 receptor in your bowel might ease irritable bowel syndrome.

What does ECS do for us?

The endocannabinoid system is involved in regulating several key aspects which contribute to our wellbeing and homeostatic balance:

- Sleep

- Mood regulations such as anxiety and depression

- Appetite stimulation or suppression

- Learning and memory, and erasing of traumatic memory.

- Pain perception

- Reproduction and fertility.

This has all been known for thousands of years. The ancient Egyptians used cannabis for inflammation, the Akkadians used it for depression, Pliny used it for gout, and Helen of Troy served it to soldiers for post-traumatic stress, where it was known as "no-grief". Even our dear Queen Victoria used it for menstrual pain.

The ECS regulates our stress and fear response

The endocannabinoid system regulates our fear and anxiety responses, as well as our stress-coping reactions. One of the major roles of this system in the brain is to assuage excessive anxiety responses helping to support our resilience to stress.

Emotions such as stress, fear and anxiety are generated in our brain in response to real or perceived danger. Our brain, which weighs only 2% of the body, consumes about 20% of our energy, and as you already know, the brain is rich in energy producing mitochondria, which are covered in CB1 receptors.[3] Thus our brain mitochondria are part of the endocannabinoid system, and therefore directly affected by stress.

Anxiety, fear and stress place high energy demands on the brain, which means that there is an increased demand for the mitochondria to produce those ATP energy packets, and so it is clear that when we are chronically stressed, our mitochondria are really going to feel it. If you remember that stress distorts the mitochondria, so it makes sense that stress is going to affect the CB1 receptors located on the mitochondrial membrane. Indeed, stress does induce prominent and sustained changes in the endocannabinoid system.[4] What is the relevance?

The endocannabinoid system is involved in fading painful memories following a traumatic event, so that with time, we are less triggered by the memories. However, the irony is that people with post-traumatic stress disorder often have fewer endocannabinoids,[5] and so the trauma can remain as vividly painful as the day it happened, even decades after the event. Of course, the stress of the perpetual trauma response has a negative impact on the endocannabinoid tone, making for a vicious cycle.

This has a wider impact because if we live in a state of heightened angst, which disrupts endocannabinoid system, the nervous system, the adrenal glands and the immune system, all of which ultimately makes us sick, tired and sad. That is no way to live.

What type of stress affects the ECS?

Anxiety is our response to future events with a degree of uncertainty such as the relentless bad news that we are fed every day on every media platform. Fear is a more acute response to something happening to you right now, such as a war or abusive situation, and post-traumatic stress disorder is when the memory/emotional experience of the traumatic event is as acute today as when it happened years ago.

Normal modern-day stressful experiences such as excessive workloads, difficult personal relationships, digital social media, or even infectious disease pandemics and the media associated with these events all contribute towards a disruption in the endocannabinoid system.[6]

Endocannabinoid deficiency syndrome

Quite likely neither you nor your doctor have heard of endocannabinoid deficiency syndrome – however, there are some symptoms associated with stress and fatigue which have been shown to be associated with endocannabinoid deficiency:[7]

- Increased sensitivity to pain, light or sound

- Migraines

- Having anxiety, depression, or trouble regulating mood

- Irregular sleep patterns or insufficient sleep

- Fibromyalgia

- Irritable bowel syndrome, or inflammatory bowel disease.

Let's add in fatigue, because we now know that the mitochondria are intimately involved in the endocannabinoid system, so our energy production is going to be impeded.

One of the most distressing symptoms of chronic fatigue syndrome is fibromyalgia. The person suffers a great amount of pain in their muscles, and yet there is no evidence of inflammation, poor blood circulation, nor spasms. The cause of the pain is a mystery. However, there is some evidence which suggests that an endocannabinoid deficiency may be a factor in fibromyalgia, as well as other conditions such as irritable bowel syndrome and migraine, where the person experiences pain, but the underlying cause remains unknown.[8]

With fibromyalgia, the pain wanders around the body as trigger points of extreme tenderness but without a known cause; this condition has been very difficult to treat. Nevertheless, there is a well-known association between fibromyalgia and chronic fatigue syndrome, adrenal fatigue, depression and anxiety, which gives us a clue.

Chronic fatigue syndrome and adrenal fatigue are associated with stress, and depression and anxiety are stress responses. We have seen above that stress has a profound effect on the endocannabinoid system, which is responsible for regulating our perception of pain and balancing our mood.

These conditions of irritable bowel syndrome, migraine headaches, fibromyalgia, anxiety, depression and insomnia are all associated with an increased perception of pain, or hypersensitivity. For instance, those who suffer from migraines will often have a strong aversion to light and sound, while those with irritable bowel syndrome feel the normal bowel stretch to be excruciatingly painful.

Because the endocannabinoid system regulates our pain perception, those with endocannabinoid deficiency are likely to suffer from conditions involving increased pain perception, or maybe mood disorders.

Using CBD products

Now the big question is: how do we repair or rebalance this vast, complicated and subtle system? It is tempting for me to elaborate on methods to repair your own endocannabinoid system, because ultimately, that is what you want – a healthy, fully functioning system without relying on external substances. However, when you are wracked with pain from fibromyalgia, or curled up in a ball with anxiety, or exhausted because you can't sleep, you are not in a position to repair own system. You need help. So let's turn to this amazing plant, *Cannabis sativa*.

The reason why most people say that they smoke cannabis is to relax, and the plant does that very well. However, the active molecule tetrahydrocannabinol (THC) is not legal in this country, and has consequences on mental health. The hemp plant contains almost no THC, but possibly hundreds of other cannabinoids.

The other cannabinoids do not make you high, yet can also be deeply relaxing, or pain relieving. The full name for the famous CBD is cannabidiol, but CBD is only one of many cannabinoids found in the plant. The other cannabinoids are like a rearrangement of the alphabet with names like CBDA, CBG, CBC, as well as terpenes and flavonoids. Even though most of these cannabinoids are found in miniscule quantities in the hemp plant, they work together as a team, known as the "entourage effect", providing a far more effective therapeutic action than simply using a high-dose CBD isolate product. Broad-spectrum CBD contains all the cannabinoids and other molecules of the plant, except THC.

Now "full-spectrum CBD" contains all the hemp cannabinoids including some THC, but only in a tiny amount. This is perfectly legal because the maximum permitted amount is 0.2%, although many products have only 0.05% THC.

The general consensus is that full-spectrum CBD is more effective than broad spectrum, and definitely more effective than CBD isolate, but if you take too large a dose, then you might feel slightly heady. Having said that, only very small doses may be needed to be effective.

Any of the experts that I have ever asked about CBD have always emphasized starting at a low dose. CBD oil comes in different strengths, with 2% to 25% or possibly even higher CBD content, but the best way to start is with a broad-spectrum or full-spectrum, low-strength oil of 3% or 5% CBD content.

Take one drop under your tongue. You don't swallow it, just hold it in your mouth and then eventually you can swallow the saliva in your mouth, because the cannabinoids easily diffuse through the blood vessels under your tongue, straight into the bloodstream.

Don't expect results immediately, but just take it slowly, watch and wait. I have used it for people with severe pain, and it has worked after a few days absolutely magnificently. What a relief it is to be out of pain. You can let go, sleep, rest and start to recover, and the joy of life returns.

It is worth making a list of your symptoms, because I cannot tell you how often I have had this experience where my patients think my herbal prescriptions have not done very much for them, until I enquire about one or other symptoms, and then their face lights up. It is such a funny thing, but when the pain goes, we just forget all about it. So do monitor your progress.

These products have been shown to benefit those with rheumatoid arthritic pain, muscle spasms, anxiety, irritable bowel syndrome, migraine headaches, fibromyalgia, post-traumatic stress disorder, Parkinson's disease, Crohn's disease, cancer-related nausea and sleep disorders, amongst others.

Restoring our own ECS

The words often found on the web are "endocannabinoid tone". This term refers to how well your endocannabinoid system is functioning, and of course, we strive to optimize our endocannabinoid tone.

Of course, when you are so fatigued, stressed out and your body is filled with pain, it is not reasonable to expect that you can somehow optimize this tone on your own. This is where the cannabinoids discussed above are very helpful. However, our body is very delicately balanced chemically, and when you provide a certain hormone or neurotransmitter, the body stops bothering to produce its own, or it shuts down some of the receptors because there are possibly more chemicals in the blood than is required. This is why it is so difficult to come off anti-depressants, because your body has adjusted to being fed chemicals which keep the serotonin in your bloodstream, and thus it doesn't make its own, plus receptors are closed down.

So in the case of cannabinoids and your own endocannabinoid system, my suggestion is to take them to get better, and then look after your own endocannabinoid system with your lifestyle choices.

The number one way to repair your endocannabinoid system is to live calmly. Life is always going to be stressful, but it is our response to life which dictates whether we thrive or stagger. Find a way to access your inner calm, your inner sanctuary of peace.

Hempseed oil

The two major endocannabinoids in our body, (anandamide and 2-arachidonoylglycerol) are made from omega-6 and omega-3 fatty acids.[9] The ideal dietary ratio of these fatty acids is constantly argued over, but on average, health experts agree that the ratio of omega-6 and omega-3 should be 3:1. Incredibly, hempseed oil naturally has exactly that ratio of omegas. Hempseed oil is not suitable for frying, but with a soft nutty taste, it is delicious to use as a salad dressing, in soups, or dip some good quality bread into it as a snack.

Chocolate

Most of us roll our eyes in bliss when we enjoy a good quality chocolate, and guess what? Chocolate has that endocannabinoid bliss chemical, anandamide, but only in tiny quantities. However, it contains two other chemicals which both activate the endocannabinoid receptors as well as inhibit the breakdown of anandamide. However, the ancient Olmecs, Mayans and Aztecs always included chilli and or vanilla in their chocolate drinks – why? Together these ingredients stimulate the production, and prevent the breakdown of, our own anandamide,[10] our own endocannabinoid of bliss. Why not try this chocolate drink to support your own endocannabinoid tone. In my recipe, I have included black pepper, chilli, nutmeg and vanilla because these work synergistically with the cacao to enhance our endocannabinoid tone.[11] [12]

 Endocannabinoid chocolate drink

½ cup of water
½ cup of your chosen milk
1 heaped tsp of raw cacao powder
A hearty pinch of chilli flakes
A pinch of freshly ground pepper
A tiny pinch of nutmeg
½ tsp of vanilla extract, or a drop of vanilla
   essence
Stevia or xylitol to sweeten

Bring to a rising boil in a pan, then pour into your cup.

Cannabinoid massage

Whilst there is debate as to whether touch or gentle massage enhances the endocannabinoid tone, most people can attest to the sense of bliss that we gain from a therapeutic massage or even gentle stroking from a loved one. Certain essential oils have been shown to enhance endocannabinoid tone of our bodies, and these are worth including if you are going to have a massage.

Although hempseed oil may only have trace amounts of cannabinoids, it makes an excellent carrier oil for essential oils which will interact with the endocannabinoid receptors on the fascia covering our muscles.[13]

Below is a short list of essential oils which have a beneficial effect on our endocannabinoid tone, and may be included in a massage oil to comfort both the mind and the body.

- Lavender (*Lavendula angustifolia*) (influences CB2)
  – anti-anxiety and pain relieving

- Cedarwood (*Cedrus atlantica*) (influences CB1 and CB2)
  – anti-anxiety and pain relieving

- Ylang-ylang (*Cananga odorata*) (influences CB2)
  – anti-depressant, relaxing, uplifting

- Copaiba oil (*Copaifera spp.*) (influences CB2)
  – peaceful, calming essential oil with anti-inflammatory pain-relieving qualities.[14]

Practices such as meditation, mindfulness, yoga and spending time in nature are daily practices that we can adopt to support our endocannabinoid tone. There are other more stringent methods, such as running which gives that "runners high", or hot and cold therapy, which you can include into your shower ritual by ending with a minute of cold water. And there are other ways too . . .

Did you know that dreams come true?

Yes, indeed they do. It is just that our brain is predisposed to be vigilant for danger, and so we tend to focus on what's going wrong, and we miss all those little things that we have wished for, and that have aligned themselves into our lives. To focus on what is wrong is to miss such an opportunity to be joyful and grateful, and thus, naturally reducing stress because you can't be stressed and grateful in the same moment. It's impossible. By focusing on gratitude and the beauties in our lives (and there are many), your mind gives your physiology the right environment to rebalance the endocannabinoid system, because as we all know – the mind and the body are one.

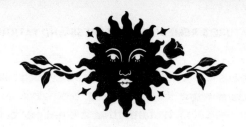

CHAPTER 13

CHANGE YOUR MIND

The sciences of quantum biophysics and epigenetics have deepened our understanding of the mind–body–spirit connection. For hundreds of years, the paradigm of Western medicine determined that the body is akin to a machine. The body belonged to medicine, and the mind/spirit belonged to the Church. Organ parts were repaired mechanistically – bits break down, the surgeon fixes them, or you take a pill to suppress the symptoms of the broken-down system, and off you go. Medicine today still pretty much adheres to this model, but in our hearts, we know that our mind and body are one. The underlying precept of holistic healing is that we are not simply a collection of body parts but a whole self-regulating system, like the Earth. All we have to do is provide the right environment for the mind/body to self-regulate.

Scientists like Rupert Sheldrake (*Morphic Resonance*, Park Street Press, 2009) have been illuminating our understanding not only of our mind–body connection, but also our interconnectedness with each other and animals. Our pets know when we are coming home long before

What the brain perceives, the mind interprets and reflects as the state of the body.

they could possibly hear the car driving down the street, and we all know that sense of being stared at, or answering the phone to someone you have just thought about. We are all interconnected.

Epigenetics is a relatively new science which reveals how our conscious state influences our biological functioning, health and wellbeing. It states, that it is not our genes which make us ill, but our response to our environment which flicks certain genes on or off, and thereby determines whether we live in poor health or wellness. That is a big statement, so how exactly does this affect you and me?

It means that by changing our mind, we can change our lived experience, and our health. If you are reading this book, you have decided to empower yourself by taking responsibility for your health. Everything that you ever achieved started in your mind, with a decision to "do something about it".

I do understand that me saying that your health is determined by your mind might be very annoying, but please do read on, because you will soon see how your conscious state can determine your wellbeing at the deepest level. Now we are diving deeply into your sense of self-empowerment, how you can change your life, and perhaps help to change the world for the better.

The biology of belief

Bruce Lipton (*The Biology of Belief*, Hay House, 2005) is one of my favourite scientists. As a biologist, he took life down to microscopic level by observing stem cells in a petri dish. We have been taught that we are powerless over our biology because our genes determine our biology. In other words, that that we are victims of our genetics. What Lipton discovered in his laboratory challenged the medical community.

In 1967, he was growing genetically identical stem cells in petri dishes. He would place a cell in a growth medium and in about 10 hours that cell divided into two identical cells. Ten hours after that there are four cells, and so on until at the end of the week he had 50,000 identical cells.

So, the cells were genetically identical and continued to be identical, until one day, he slightly changed the chemicals in the growth medium of each dish. To his surprise, in one petri dish the cells produced muscle tissue, in the next bone tissue, and the next produced fat cells. At that moment, Bruce Lipton realized that it was not the genetics of the cells which determined the destiny of the cell, but the environment. The cells were all identical but the environment in which they were growing had changed, and in response to the environment, the cells had changed. At this point, you might say, well, so what?

But, human beings are not a single entity. We are a community of about 50 trillion cells, plus another 100 trillion bacteria which live in our guts. In our bodies, instead of the cells being cultured within a liquid medium held by a petri dish, our skin is the petri dish, and our cells are nourished by the growth medium of our blood.

Our blood provides the environment in which our cells grow, but who controls the blood chemistry? It is the hormones which are the chemicals in our blood, and where do these hormones come from? They are produced by messages from our brain. What is it that stimulates which hormones are released from our brain? This is down to our outlook on life.

If you see love and joy in the world, then your brain interprets that image and responds by releasing dopamine, oxytocin and growth hormone – the hormones of love and health. We all know that those people who feel love and joy glow with vitality.

However, if that same person looks out at the world from a fearful perspective, the brain is going to release stress hormones such as adrenaline and cortisol. As you know, these hormones do not produce vibrant health but instead depress our immune system and trigger inflammation, predisposing us to becoming ill.

If you interpret the world in a positive way, you release chemicals that enhance vital health and you open up to the world. If you are anxious or stressed, you naturally want to protect yourself and hide from the world. This is relevant to health because you can't be open and closed at the same time. You cannot be anxious and stressed, and yet be in a state of wellness because your blood chemistry will be secreting hormones of stress, not vitality. If you maintain a positive outlook on life, your brain releases hormones which support excellent immunity, healing and repairing of old cells, and thus maintains your state of vital health.

Depending on our choice of mindset, we can change the chemicals in our blood, which influences which gene will be expressed, and that determines our health. What you see or believe is translated by your mind into the chemistry which controls the functioning of your cells, and thus, your health. We are the conductor of the orchestra of our body. It is our brain, our consciousness and our belief which determines our health.

Of course, if you look at mainstream media – it is all about fear, shock and horror. Hideous stuff. Detach yourself from that rubbish and look at the flowers. Look at nature, the beauty of the skies, wisdom of trees, the love that shines from your dog or friend's eyes, listen to the birds singing, go singing yourself. In this way you nourish the growth medium in your body by triggering healthy hormones which will support life. In this way, you take back your power and your vital health.

The cell mem-brain

Now here is something even more interesting. The intelligence of a cell is determined by the surface area of the membrane because it is the cell membrane which interfaces between the internal environment of the cell and the external environment in which it is living. It is the membrane of the cell which determines what is absorbed and excreted, it instructs the cells to move towards nutrition and away from toxins. So the membrane is the "brain" of the cell.

We know that we have evolved from bacteria. A single bacteria only has a certain amount of membrane surface area, and so when it has realized its full potential because of the limitation of the amount of surface area on its membrane, it has two choices: it can either stop developing at that point, or can join with other bacteria to share a greater surface area of membrane, and continue to develop as a communal entity. Through evolution, different bacteria joined communally, and shared their different membrane intelligences and resources, until they integrated to become multi-cellular organisms. At some stage in their evolution these organisms reach their maximum ability to develop, and larger multi-cellular organisms were formed, finally evolving into human beings. That is what we are – 50 trillion cells, a community of cells developed from bacteria.

Now we have reached the zenith of where we can evolve to as humans (hence we have artificial intelligence), and you can see from this trajectory of evolution that our pathway will insist that we learn to join up with others and recognize that we are a community of humans. Much more than that, we are a community of cells living on planet Earth. We are the cells of Gaia, along with the other cells, which are the trees, the herbs, the waters, the soil, the animals. We are all one, and of course, that is the consciousness that is emerging now. We cannot save ourselves if we don't save our environment, which is our ultimate growth medium. The way that we can join the evolutionary leap is by joining up with other people, so that we have a sense of belonging, shared resources, and where we protect the natural world. Understandably you may be wondering what this has to do with stress and fatigue.

There are certain communities in the world where an unusually large proportion of people live in vibrant health way into their 90s or even well over 100. These pockets of exceptionally long-lived humans are healthy, full of joy and vitality. One of the strongest commonalities between these societies is that they have strong community bonds, which engender feelings of security and laughter and love, and this is the exact mindset needed to generate those health-giving hormones in our bloodstream.

So, let's have a look at some of these communities and see what they are doing to live so well.

Blue Zone

In the late 21st C, an adventurer and leader of expeditions called Dan Buettner (*The Blue Zones*, National Geographic, 2012) set out to find the areas of the world where people generally live longer than average. He had travelled widely, and was clearly a man with an intense curiosity about people and cultures. On a map of the world he circled five "longevity hotspot" areas in blue, which became known as The Blue Zones.

While chronic disease is becoming increasingly common in the developed world, these Blue Zones communities experience low rates of chronic disease and live in good health, easily into their 90s. He also confirms – genetics only accounts for about 20–30% of our longevity and ability to live well. The rest is determined by our lifestyle and our diet.

The five Blue Zones

Ikaria (Greece): a tiny island in the Greek archipelago, where the residents ignore the clock, take a short afternoon nap, and incorporate exercise into their lifestyles as they grow their vegetables. They enjoy late-night dominoes and red wine with their island friends.

Ogliastra, Sardinia (Italy): the Ogliastra region of Sardinia is home to the greatest concentrations of men who live to be over 100 in the world. This rugged mountainous area hosts tight family values where the residents have low rates of depression. Grandparents are celebrated and actively contribute to society. Their diet centres around what they hunt and grow, with an accent on vegetables and goat's milk. They too have a strong sense of community where they gather in the streets and bars in the afternoon to laugh with their friends and enjoy red wine.

Okinawa (Japan): the islands at the southern end of Japan are known as the "land of the immortals". Here we have a group of the world's longest-living women. It is a community which lives by a centuries-old system called a "maoi", where as part of their culture they develop lifelong friendships which provide a network of social, financial, spiritual and health support. In the villages, these friends meet daily or weekly to share stories and advice, to pool resources and even offer financial support if it is needed.

They also practise a concept called *ikigai*, which translates into "a reason for being", or a sense of purpose. It is that feeling of satisfaction which comes from pursuing your passion. In Okinawa, many elderly people have an *ikigai*, such as friends, gardening or art.

Nicoya Peninsula (Costa Rica): the folk in these communities also naturally incorporate into their life a reason for living, known as "plan de vida": that which gives their life purpose and drives a buoyant outlook on life. They have strong community ties, and enjoy physical work well into their very old age.

The Seventh-day Adventists in Loma Linda, California are a close-knit religious community who view health as being central to their faith. They eat a mainly vegetarian diet, and once a week take a day to pray, focus on nature and their community. They also give back to their community and therefore have a sense of purpose and belonging.

Blue Zone commonalities

Generally, it was found that these strong people from different cultures around the world had a few lifestyle patterns in common:

- **They integrate movement into their lifestyles.**

They are moving at a natural human pace, rather than whizzing around at breakneck speed exhausting themselves. Instead of sweating it out at the gym, they grow their gardens, sweep their homes without electrical conveniences, walk with their goats over rugged terrain, and walk rather than drive to visit their friends.

What can we do?

We can manage our own gardens or allotments, or help someone who isn't able to manage their garden. Growing our own food provides far more nutrition than shop-bought food. Vitamin C degrades rapidly after harvest with up to 77% lost within three days of harvest. When you grow your own vegetables, you really can taste the difference.

Collect your own wood for your wood burners, cut it and store it for winter. Wild harvest your blackberries and elderberries for winter health tonics. Get to know your rural landscape by walking the land, if possible, with friends, and take time to stop for a drink or have a picnic along the way.

- **They nurture strong bonds.**

Long-lived communities put their loved ones first, investing time and energy in spending quality time with the older and younger members of their families. Blue Zone people spend a lot of time with their family, friends and loved ones just hanging out, maybe drinking wine, maybe fishing, maybe drinking tea and probably chatting about everyone else! Almost all of the Blue Zone people mention laughing a lot.

What can we do?

Family does not have to just be blood relations. You can create a family through close bonds and regular contact with any group of people, such as knitting circles, drumming circles, communal vegetable growing, mothers groups, helping our neighbours. These are people that you can feel safe with, who support you and are supported by you. No person is an island, and strong bonds create that vital support network. Sharing loving relationship with life-long friends or family also increases quality of life as traditions are created, and rituals of care for each other are created with events to look forward. Make sure that being with these people makes you feel good, and that you laugh a lot.

- **They take time out every day.**

Just being alive is stressful. It doesn't matter where you are in the world, you worry about your crops failing, sudden accidents, your children's future, and everything else that life throws at you. We have to accept that there is always going to be stress, but the key is how we manage our stress. In the Blue Zones, these folk take a stress-free break every day according to their tradition. Some spend time in meditation or prayer, whilst others take an afternoon siesta, and some meet their friends at the bar after fishing.

What can we do?

Join a yoga class, walk in the country, practise meditation, mindfulness or spending time in your sacred zone. You might like to do something that puts you into the state of flow. Whatever it is, it is time for your brain and/or your body to rest.

- **They have a purpose in their lives.**

They have a reason to wake up in the morning. They have purpose in their lives, a reason to get up in the morning because there is something in their lives that really matters to them. They are not just old redundant people. Their purpose often involves a service to others. This gives their life meaning.

Viktor Frankl (*Man's Search for Meaning*, Rider Press, 2021) wrote that "He who has a why to live for, can bear with almost any how." Frankl was a Jewish psychiatrist who lived through the concentration camps of the Holocaust. During his years in those death camps, he found that if a person had a reason to live, then he would find a way to do it, no matter how difficult. Those with a reason or purpose tend to live longer and better.

What can we do?

The most prevalent reason for living is something that you deeply care about, and usually involves giving back to society. You might focus on your family, or animal rescue, or perhaps you manage the local village hall, or are writing a self-help book, taking the grandchildren home from school and helping with their after-school care, restoring an ancient building, creating a communal vegetable garden, or you may be a mentor for some group such as Alcoholics Anonymous where you are helping people to live their best lives with the help of your life experience.

• **Eat lightly.**

Most Blue Zone diets occasionally include meat, but mostly they live on beans and legumes, vegetables, seasonal fruits, but very little refined carbohydrates. These folk cook from scratch and they eat together in a leisurely manner. They also tend to stick to the "80% rule", which is that they stop eating when they feel 80% full, and tend to eat earlier in the evening.

What can we do?

When we are stressed or over busy, we tend to bolt our food down, without even tasting it, and certainly not paying any attention to how we feel as we eat it. I love that Buddhist saying to your foo... take time to sav... and really appreciate ... f life's great pleasures, so do ... In other words, pay attention to enjoy. Eating slowly a...e. Show your food respect less because it gives your bra... at you have the privilege stomach is satisfied. ...sly will result in eating ... to register that your

There is a huge difference in ten... calorie intake between eating until you are full, and ea... until you are not hungry. Eating lightly keeps you light, and ...s has major benefits on our ability to move easily, and live comfo...ably.

- **They enjoy a glass or two.**

People in all Blue Zones (except Adventists) drink alcohol moderately and regularly, enjoying 1 – 2 glasses of wine per day with friends and food. Moderate drinking seems to have a protective effect on the cardiovascular system, and they live longer.

- **They have balance in their lives.**

I think it is also important to point out that some people's energy is enhanced by being with others, whilst other people need time on their own. You will have to find your own balance according to how much time you need alone versus with people, but you can still have strong bonds around you even if you are one of those who needs more time alone. Myself, I need time alone but I also love being with people. On weekday evenings, and sometimes even for an entire weekend, I need time in silence and alone because that is how I find my balance. I am invigorated by a walk in the hills or along the hedgerows, a happy chat with neighbours, or meditating in the monastery, but I don't always engage in deep and meaningful conversations because I do that all week and I need to just "be".

NATURE'S REMEDIES F...

Some of us like to work ...

others prefer to work f...

matter. What matters ...

but it is always abou...

some time for your...

then do some phy...

group where you...

and have fun. A...

you without giv...

get enough ...

Really...

...y companies, whilst either way it does not do what is right for you – If you work very hard, take y day. If your job is very mental, ercise. If you are a carer, then join a lk about yourself. Take your holidays ose who draw too much energy from back. Make sure you eat a balanced diet, st, enough outdoor fun time, enough love. try to reconnect with nature – it is the greatest re-balancer of all.

Energies are contagious

Choose your words wisely for they will become who you are. Your subconscious mind is absolutely amazing, and it remembers every single thing that you have ever experienced. This part of our mind works in feelings and not words, and the more you reiterate a feeling or experience, the more that becomes imprinted on the subconscious. It becomes your learned belief which is expressed by who you become.

The words that you use are extremely powerful because they all carry a particular feeling frequency. Every time you see or hear certain words, the subconscious notices. Eventually it believes. The child who is told that they will never make anything of themselves, manifests just that. Elvis Presley was born in the poorest part of town, in the poorest state of America, but his mother instilled in him the belief that he was destined for greatness, and he became one of the most loved men ever to walk this earth. He became "The King". Words have energy. His power, by the way, was not his voice or his gyrations, it was the love that he radiated wherever he went. Love has power beyond anything else and energies are contagious.

Our mind is divided into the conscious and the subconscious mind. Our conscious mind is the clever one which quickly learns that we want to get well and that we are worthy of love, and that we deserve a fulfilling life, but it only has a 5% influence on our final decision making. The real power lies in the subconscious, which learns very slowly but governs 95% of your decisions and how you respond to life. In the first seven years of your life your subconscious absorbed everything it perceived. It believed everything, and these beliefs became the landscape of your mind, because your subconscious does not change its mind unless it learns to through repetition or therapeutic modality such as hypnotherapy.

This consolidation of learned beliefs continues throughout our lives unless we make a concerted and conscious effort to repeatedly use words and pay attention to thoughts which are supportive to our health landscape.

Do you see that we are not just fixing body parts here, we are healing holistically, and that encompasses creating healthy mental pathways, influencing which hormones are secreted, and those in turn create health and wellbeing.

Dr Masaru Emoto (*Hidden Messages in Water*, Atria Books, 2005) demonstrated how water crystals respond to words which carry emotional resonance. He showed how a word such as "hate" produced a sludgy distorted crystal, whilst a word like "love" produce a beautiful snowflake-shaped crystal. On average, 66% of our physical body is made up of water, so you can imagine the powerful effect that the energy of words has on the waters within our bodies. Every cell in our body is a sac filled with intracellular fluid, so the words have an effect on our very cells, generating healthy or unhealthy patterns.

Try this for yourself by tuning into the word "uncertainty" and see how you feel. When I do that, I feel slightly shaky inside and insecure. Now try "contentment" and see how you feel. I feel safe, strong and uplifted.

The media have bandied around the word "uncertainty" since 9/11, and guess what? Everybody is anxious these days. During the Covid period, I was one of the few calm people that I knew because I don't have a television and don't buy a newspaper. I won't buy into all that scare-mongering. There are better things to think about.

There is no doubt that we pick up energies from people and our environment. We all know that sense of being stared at from behind, which clearly proves that we are all able to pick up on the energies without even trying. Rupert Sheldrake wrote a book about it called *The Sense of Being Stared at*, (Arrow Books, 2004). He shows us that our perceptive abilities are stronger than we are generally aware of.

Quantum physics has a famous experiment which demonstrates that observation actually changes the behaviour of electrons. The atoms in our body are made up of electrons. Thus if our attention has a measurable effect on our electrons, naturally the atoms and cells in our body cannot help but respond to the effect of that attention.

So we must be very careful about where we place our attention. The company you keep, the books you read, the films that you watch all require your attention, and therefore become part of your mental environment. This is terribly important, because we are influenced by and ultimately become that environment. We cannot help absorbing and reflecting the energies that surround and interpenetrate us, which will either heal or disturb us.

We live in a very strange world where violence and degradation are glamorized, but you can choose carefully what you watch and what you read, saturating your consciousness with kindness and positive beliefs. These

Choose carefully, for your environment will become you.

healing energies will embed into your subconscious mind and create a positive healing field in your mental environment which will be expressed in your physical wellbeing.

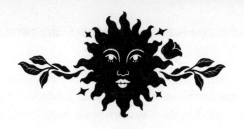

CHAPTER 14

STAYING WELL

Over the years of helping people to recover from chronic fatigue due to various causes, many conversations have resulted in a few key points pertaining to the healing journey which I would like to share with you.

Instant balance

One of the most immediate and significant things you can do for your health and to restore balance is to keep your blood sugars even. Most (if not all) highly stressed people have very erratic eating patterns and therefore erratic blood sugar levels. This leave you with very little feeling of secure stamina. If you avoid breakfast, your blood sugars will be low, then maybe you have coffee and a croissant, and it swings sharply up and you can take on the world, but the insulin kicks in, and down the blood sugars plummet again. Because you are too busy, you only notice when you are becoming irritable with tiredness, so you eat a sandwich of poor nutritional value, and up your blood sugars go again, swinging up and down throughout the day. Very erratic, exhausting and unsustainable.

By eating small quantities of highly nutritious food throughout the day you will find that you immediately feel on much more solid ground. That very day, your body will feel calmer because it is no longer dealing with swinging blood sugars and trying to cope with cortisol levels shooting up due to low blood sugar. You will be feeding your cells with nutrients that can be used to heal your body, and by not over-burdening your digestive system with large meals, the gut is able to easily digest and absorb these nutrients. In this way you are treating your body with respect – and you will feel the benefits immediately.

The trick to maintaining this programme is by being organized. Get the food that you need into your home so that it is readily available, and you'll be amazed at how much stronger, calmer and in control you feel.

Guard your energy

This happens almost invariably with my patients. They have been ill for some time, and are deeply frustrated that they can't get on with the things that they want to do. So naturally, as soon as a bit of energy starts to grow, they are off, like a racehorse at the starting gate, whizzing around doing things. Inevitably there is a crash, and then great fear that all that had been gained is now lost.

The recovery that you have made is not lost if you look after it carefully. In the early stages it is very fragile, and while you can enjoy it, you must be very careful not to abuse your energy levels. If you do abuse your energy, you will relapse, but a little stepping over the mark and a little relapse is normal and nothing will be lost. If you have a relapse, do not panic. Just go back to doing what you have been doing, and then be a little more careful with your energy next time, and you will recover. Gradually your energy will grow.

I always say to my patients that recovery is like the housing market, it goes up and down, but the general trajectory is up. Two steps forward, one step back – it's a dance.

At first, you may only have a few hours where you suddenly realize that you feel "normal", and then the fatigue comes back. If you nurture yourself, you will find that you have another few hours, and then half a day, and then a few days, until in the main, you feel well all the time.

Over time, if you look after yourself, most people are able to live as if they are perfectly healthy again, but there is one caveat. You will always have to guard your energies. For instance, yesterday I spoke to Lyn, who is just starting to turn a corner in her fatigue recovery. She was able to go out the day before and enjoy herself, but when she got home, she needed to have a little lie-down. The next day she had a very gentle day at home. Further down the track, when you feel well most of the time, if you feel your energies flagging, then take time out. Go to bed early for a few nights with a special book and be cosy in your own space.

Drains and radiators

The company that we keep does have an influence on our wellbeing. There are those who will drain you, and others who energize you. If you can't avoid the drains, try to limit your contact by keeping it brief and friendly. When you feel dread at the idea of spending time with someone, that person is a drain for you. S/he may not necessarily be a drain for anyone else, but somehow your energies are sucked away when you spend too much time with that person. It isn't their fault, they won't have a clue that they have that effect on you, so you diplomatically keep your boundaries. Usually if you explain to people that you haven't felt well for some time and that you can only cope with a short visit, they understand. If they won't understand, then you know what you have to do.

The radiators might be people who you had never imagined were the true friends that they really are, and these are people to cherish.

You cannot protect yourself and thrive at the same time.

When professor of biology Bruce Lipton (*The Biology of Belief*) studied the behaviour of human stem cells in his petri dishes, he couldn't help noticing that when nutrition was introduced to the dish of live cells, the cells gravitated towards the nutrients, allowing them to grow and thrive. However, when a poisonous substance was introduced to the live cells, the cells moved away, and in order to protect themselves, the cells had to shut down all the portals to their interior environment, to wall themselves off from the toxic environment. They turned themselves into miniature citadels.

At this point, Lipton made a very exciting connection: the cells were not able to concurrently thrive *and* defend themselves at the same time. In order to grow, they needed to open their channels to the nutrient-rich environment, but in order to protect themselves from the toxic environment, they had to close all channels. They couldn't be open and closed at the same time. The cells could either protect themselves or thrive, but could not do both at the same time. This, he noted, is exactly like our human existence, in that you cannot protect yourself and thrive at the same time. You can protect yourself and survive for a while, but you can't thrive in such an environment.

In our human situation and in the social context within which we live, we cannot expect to thrive when we are constantly having to protect ourselves from a stressful environment. Humans, animals and plants only grow and thrive in an environment which is nurturing. We wither, and parts of us die when we live on junk food and in an environment of unkindness.

Do consider your own life – whether there are any physical or mental environments, dietary choices, or habits which are metaphorically or literally poisonous to you. Could you live more robustly if you departed from these environments and moved towards a more wholesome choice?

Pacing

Our ancient ancestors, and indeed those few societies who still live an indigenous life, did not spend their time racing around doing things non-stop. They carefully planned, say, a hunt, put a lot of energy into that hunt, and then sat around for a while carving tools, etc. Even our grandmothers always took life at a far more leisurely pace than we do. They would do their chores, but there was always time to sit down with a neighbour for a cuppa and a natter.

You have choices.

Probably even less than ten years ago, graded exercise was a major component of a chronic fatigue recovery programme. It rarely worked because this is not an illness of poor conditioning, although with time, of course, the muscles do weaken. Now, graded exercise has been debunked, and pacing is the name of the game, where you do a little, then rest a little.

I use the analogy of a bank account, and when I start to see someone, s/he usually has very little in their energy bank account, so we need to build it up. It always happens this way, but as soon as a little energy returns to the person, they joyfully whizz around doing all the things that they have been longing to do, and then guess what? Relapse and despair.

So I tell my patients that they must always try to keep some energy currency in their bank account. As an example, you might decide to go on a shopping trip with your mum or sister, which is great. But as soon as you start to feel weary (please note, not when you feel bone weary and ready to collapse), you sit down, have a little snack and a cup of tea. Perhaps you will feel ready to continue your shopping trip, or perhaps that is enough for the day. This setting of energy boundaries, of course with consideration for those who accompany you, becomes a healthy lifetime habit.

I have come to the conclusion that our bodies are wiser than our minds. Our minds want to do this, and then that, and after that, then something else. Our body says, "Thank you, that was wonderful but I need to rest now." If you don't obey your body, trust me, inevitably it will make you stop, so it is worth striking a compromise between your body and your mind, which is where pacing comes into it.

Listen to your body

The body is wiser than the mind. The body will be desperate for a rest, but the mind will insist that something needs to be done, or that we must stay to the last minute of the party. The will-power usually overrules the body, until the body rebels.

I have noticed over the years that especially those who have CFS/ME or adrenal burn-out, these people are the type of person who never stop. They are the people who are perfectionists, who need to finish just one more task before they will allow themselves to stop, and they just keep going. As a result, they have learned to ignore, and then become completely deaf to, that message from their body begging for rest.

The vast majority of chronically fatigued people that I have helped have told me that allowing themselves time to rest, or to be looked after, is one of the hardest things to get their head around. They work so hard at looking after everyone else, and have an overwhelming fear of being thought of as lazy or not pulling their weight. One woman told me how she lies in bed every night aching with fatigue, but still will not stop rushing about.

I explain to people that they have become deaf to their own needs, and they need to re-learn how to hear and honour their inner message of "I need to rest". Whereas they would usually ignore the message, sending another one back to themselves saying "I just have to finish this job" or "I don't have time to rest", now I urge them to immediately obey the message. The very minute you perceive the message "I am starting to feel a little tired now", you must do everything you can to stop what you are doing and sit down. You need to remind yourself that it is entirely possible to continue with the job in half an hour's time. Give yourself permission to take life at a more measured pace. Shall we say, at a saner pace?

If this is too difficult, it might be easier for you to schedule into your daily routine a mid-morning rest for half an hour, a proper lunch break and a mid-afternoon rest of half an hour. This is not time to look at your emails, or do the bills. This is time when you relax and enjoy your rest. Go outside and lie in the sun, or snuggle on the sofa with the cat for a little while. This rest period will help to build your energy, and you will find that you can achieve just as much, but with less of that aching fatigue at the end of the day, and, this is very important . . . by treating yourself with respect, you teach your children that it is okay to live at a humane pace of life.

I have met so many people who say that their mother used to be doing the ironing at 10 o'clock at night. Well, that is just mad. We are powerfully influenced by our parental models but if the model is making you unwell, you have to redefine a new model for yourself.

> **Give yourself permission to take life at a more measured pace.**

Soothe your inner perfectionist with thoughts of gentleness towards yourself rather than obeying the inner tyrant. Be kind to yourself. Let others be kind to you too. Perhaps you are reading this and thinking to yourself – "Well that is all very well, but I work and have a family to care for. I haven't got the time." This brings us to the next major step that you can take to help bring balance back into your life.

Let others help you

People with chronic fatigue tend to be very independent. This may be either because they dare not ask for help, or they do not have a partner, or in most cases because they will not allow their family and friends to help them.

Recently I asked a very busy and completely exhausted lady if she ever allows her partner to help her and she said that she does not. When I asked her how she thinks he feels about this, she suddenly burst into tears saying that he feels pushed out. This was a very important moment for this lady because she suddenly realized that he wants to help her.

It would make him feel useful being able to protect and care for the woman he loves. By not allowing herself to rest and be cared for, she continues flogging the proverbial nearly-dead horse, making her partner feel redundant and powerless. By insisting on doing it all herself, she denies him the joy of demonstrating how much he loves her.

I am not saying that you should lie on your bed and do nothing for months, although some people are so ill with exhaustion that that is all they can do. This lady will continue to work, but perhaps her partner will make supper whilst she relaxes in the bath, and she will allow him to fetch the kids or bring her a cup of tea on the sofa, so that she can allow her body to recover.

If you really insist that there are jobs to do which cannot be ignored, and you cannot bear to ask your family to do them, perhaps you could pay someone to do your ironing or cleaning, or discuss with your boss that you need an assistant, or reduce your hours.

People love to help those they love, so please let your loved ones help you. Don't be afraid to ask, and don't feel guilty. It will make them feel good, develop a lovely sense of togetherness, and bring to you a warm feeling of being nurtured and cared for.

Follow your own path

It is generally well known that research into the psychology of those suffering with chronic fatigue syndrome shows a trend towards those who are high achievers, or those who have undergone prolonged and unacknowledged stress.

Years ago when I worked on my MSc dissertation, I wanted to understand why people suffering from ME were so frequently high achievers. These people try 110% at work or at home, they tend to be people-pleasers, and the work-hard-play-hard type. When I discussed this with my sample group of those who had suffered and recovered from ME, they consistently revealed to me that through most of their lives they had suppressed their own needs or dreams, rather following the expectations of others. They did this to gain acceptance or to feel safe and lovable. It didn't matter whether their mother actually had other expectations of her child; it was simply enough that the child believed she needed to achieve or behave in a certain manner in order to be loved. In not following their own paths in life, or over-compensating – they became people-pleasers, perfectionists or worked too hard and ultimately burnt themselves out.

Then, I asked the same people what was the turning point in their recovery from ME. They told me that it was when they finally learnt to accept themselves and followed their own needs. They followed their heart and focused on spending time with people who are good to be around, and by doing the work or hobbies that they were born to do, or that they love to do. In other words, they treat themselves with love by fulfilling their inner and unique creativity. By working like this, you work with joy, and the joy is energy-giving and healthy.

You can start to live your dream by daydreaming about what it is that you would love to do, if you were able to do it. We all came into this world with a special gift, and when we do that, it is called working in the "flow state". This is when you feel so at home with what you are doing, feel so engaged, that everything else just disappears. Flow state always stems from doing what you were born to do.

Sometimes it is hard to know what we would love to do, and if that is the case, try to remember what you fantasized about as a child, because the child is often more in touch with themselves than the adult.

Dream your dream.

Then you might argue that it is impossible, but it is amazing how things can work out if you hold a dream in your heart. You can start by just imagining how you might possibly get there, and it is just magical how opportunities open up.

Explain to people how you feel

A lot of people with fatigue find that they are highly reactive to even the smallest bit of stress and can become extremely agitated over tiny issues. This is quite understandable because they are at a place where they just cannot take any more, and in self-defence they lash out.

The problem is that this intolerance can manifest as irritability, irrational rage or a longing to get away from it all, and can be very difficult for the person to live with, and also challenging and confusing for the person's family to live with. This excessive sensitivity to stress is very stressful in itself, perpetuating the adrenal fatigue. It is better to be kind to yourself and if you are feeling particularly sensitive one day, to stay away from potentially aggravating people or situations, if at all possible, until you feel better.

Some people find that they need a lot of time alone, with sensory deprivation, to recover their ability to deal with the franticness of the world they live in. Sensory deprivation means enjoying spending time in silence, just quietly and gently pottering about. Make sure that your blood sugar levels are comfortable, because low blood sugars can make one feel even more irritable.

Bear in mind that most people don't understand this condition and are trying to be helpful, even if they sometimes go about it in a clumsy way. It can really make a difference if you explain to your family how you are feeling, and how this illness is difficult for you. Ask them to be patient with you at these times, and to give you the space and kindness that you need. Once people understand, they are usually very happy to get on board with you, because they love you and want to help you to get better.

Kind Things

When I was a child, I decided that there was a balance in life between "kind things" vs "nasty things". In order to be able to deal with life, "kind things" had to outweigh "nasty things". I have to emphasize here that I had a very nice life and was not deprived in any way, but ordinary life tasks like homework were chalked up as "nasty things". Kind things became a philosophy of life. It is a way of living which I still do, and I have to say, it serves me rather well.

"Kind things" involves anything which I consider to be self-nourishing. This might be floating in a warm fragrant bath, or planting a pretty window box outside my bedroom window, or lying under a tree and looking at the sky through the filigree twigs, cuddling the dog, a pot of tea and a good book, cycling through the park at dusk listening to the deer bellowing in the autumn, going to bed at 6pm if I feel like it, making soup from my vegetable garden, having friends round for tea and a home-made cake. Other people might like to go to the gym and then enjoy a hot steam. It really doesn't matter, as long as your mind and body recognize that you are being kind to yourself.

These little things in life matter. They rarely involve much money but they bring great pleasure. The contentment that you get from "kind things" ripples from you like an enchantment, and you find that others around you find their own "kind things". Soon your network focuses on kindness, joy and contentment instead of angst, stress and fatigue.

The gift

It may be that you feel as if your world has imploded. For hundreds of years spiritual teachers have referred to extended and particularly difficult times in our lives as the "dark night of the soul". These are not just little moments when you feel a bit sorry for yourself, but those profound times in our lives where despair cracks you open to the core, and coming through it is fundamentally life-changing. It feels as if you have survived a major emotional or spiritual earthquake – which you have. The dark night of the soul can rock you so deeply that even years afterwards, the memory can bring tears to your eyes.

I hope it doesn't sound incredibly crass to say that these can be very precious times. If you can find the wisdom to know that there is always a deeper purpose, and this is not meaningless. If you can find the courage to accept these times which will pass but will leave their mark on your soul, you will find there is a profundity to gain.

The trick is to remember that it always passes, and it leaves you changed for the better. During these times, you might want to retreat from people, and that is absolutely fine because there is an instinctive urge to be alone and reconnect with yourself. This reconnection process is the precious jewel.

Sometimes in life one has no choice but to allow yourself to sink right down to the bottom of the well, into the dark unknown depths of your despair. There you spend time amongst the tears, mud and slime which is also a part of each of us, and your hand, groping for something to hold onto, suddenly clasps a pebble. Then you will rise up through that dark well and once the waters of time have washed away the mud, you find in your hand a jewel which represents the real pure "You". You in all your pure iridescent beauty. The You who you really are, what you are capable to being, and what you have to offer the world.

The real You, drowned in the silt and mud which represent the years of conditioning to which we have all been subjected. In that mud, our true talents and destinies are put aside, forgotten and hidden from view. But if you can find within yourself the courage to drift down into the depths of yourself, and find the talent, the hobby, the vocation which makes you joyful, which fires your imagination and which makes your heart sing – then you know where to follow your own path towards a life where the real You shines so brightly again – just as you were born to do.

Each of us are born with some gift which makes us shine brightly. It is just that the vast majority of us get caught up in what we ought to be doing rather than what we were born to do. Now is the time to be true to yourself and allow your soul to shine its own unique light – so that you brighten life up a little more for the rest of us.

I have often suggested to my patients that they consider their illness as a great gift. Of course, you can imagine that they do not always respond well to this point of view, but I offer them the idea that they got to this point because of the way they lived their lives, or responded to life. If this illness can be seen as a turning point, a time when they can reconsider the way they live their lives, and a chance to re-imagine how they want to live. Perhaps you could think of the illness as a rite of passage, an opportunity to take stock and reconsider your whole life ahead – in doing so, it can be seen as the chance to transform your relationship with life into one which is life-sustaining and allows you to thrive with vigour and joy, not just survive.

Covid offered us the same gift but this time it was on a global scale. The world stopped. It was unbelievable. There was silence and even peace. People could rest, think, reconsider, many didn't go back to their old jobs again, and the world was changed forever after Covid.

Suggested Reading:
Thomas Moore, *The Dark Night of the Soul,* Piatkus, 2012

Our brain is hard-wired to worry, and this happens at all levels of life. See how the sparrows constantly look around while they eat birdseed, or the dog barks when there is a slight noise outside the door, or the cat watches every shadow at the window. It's a natural protective mechanism, but it can become overwhelming and stressful.

However, here is the irony: we need a degree of stress to feel alive and engaged in our lives. If you remember the endocrinologist, Hans Selye, at the beginning of this book, who described general adaptation syndrome to stress. He also coined the term "eustress" (eu meaning good).

Eustress occurs when we have a challenge, something that we really want, but it is out of reach, although not so out of reach that we cannot aspire to it. A valued goal. The challenge and effort that we put into attaining that goal energizes us, and brings a sense of heightened life satisfaction.

The challenge of eustress motivates us to become more than we think we can be. It gives us a sense of hope, and then the satisfaction of achieving a goal which will add value to our lives. In doing so, it actually enhances our physical and mental wellbeing. This is a very healthy stress, and one which we can all bring into our lives.

The ultimate eustress experience is when we are "in flow", or "in the zone". These are moments where we are completely absorbed in what we are doing, with no awareness of time or our surroundings. You are fully focused on attending to your challenge, and the experience

. So, it
only we can determine
of our comfort zones are, but the range is limited

It's important that you valued goal be broken down into steps which are small enough that you are not daunted, and that you can actually take those steps. Then you start to take control of your life because you are

> In moving out of your comfort zone, you actually realign more deeply with the real you.

engaging in that which you love, and becoming that which you were meant to be.

Your goal is living the life you were born to live, and not many people have the courage to do that. Most will rather live safely, within boundaries predetermined by their upbringing, and often in the state of being "happily unhappy". But if you choose to take the challenge of eustress, to strive towards your valued goal, you will be one of the few who live a life of contentment and peace, and that in itself acts as a buffer against a very stressful world.

Silver linings

What if you find yourself in a difficult situation right now? How do you get out of it? To every situation, there is always a silver lining if you are the sort of person who looks for them. The silver lining may simply be that this situation is so awful that it is forcing you to make scary life choices to change. It is kicking your butt out of the rut.

So when you find yourself in a distressing situation, try to play your life forward, and see if you can find the silver lining in the situation that you are in today. Use that silver lining as an inspiration to make different life choices. It becomes an opportunity to change your life for the better, and in doing so, you have chosen to take control rather than being controlled by your stress response. The payoff is enormous.

My hope is that you declutter your mind and strengthen your body, so that you are able to take up the challenge of your valued goal, and live your best life.

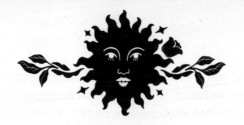

CHAPTER 16

LIFE MAPS

Usually the biggest questions on someone's mind are:

- Will I ever be healthy again?

- Can I get my life back to the way it was?

- And, how long will it take?

These are very reasonable questions to ask, but difficult for a health practitioner to answer because everyone's situation and health condition is unique. The time it takes for recovery will vary according to individual stamina reserves, the length of illness, the current conditions under which one lives, other contributing factors such as viruses or gut parasites, and of course the severity of the symptoms.

However, there is a rule of thumb in natural medicine which states that recovery takes approximately one month, for every year that you have been ill. But as you know, your health might have been under considerable strain without you realizing it for years before it actually broke down. Taking all these, and many other, variables into account, you can understand that it is difficult to make a prediction.

It is very important to look at the precipitating patterns which set you up for the breakdown of health, and then to exchange those patterns for healthier choices. Patterns which include pushing yourself too hard have probably been playing out for most of your life, and so you can see that change will not happen overnight, nor will recovery occur immediately because there is a lot of repair work to do.

You can choose another way of living which is much more sustainable. We are all talking about sustainability now. The unsustainable environmental stress under which our planet labours presents a sobering metaphor of the way people are treating their own bodies. Sucking all the oil from the earth, stripping the soil of all its nutrients, endless growth, cutting the forests down is unsustainable, and most sane people recognize that it is impossible to continue in that manner. This is the same for your own body and these types of situations insist upon change.

Taking stock

Bearing in mind that this book is concerned with the effects of stress on our health, you might want to ask yourself: "What was it that got me into this position?" Possibly there were events beyond your control, but they may still need to be attended to with counselling, or making a choice to move on in your life. It may be that you are the sort of person who looks after everyone else's needs, paying scant attention to your own, and that may need to be adjusted. Perhaps you need to reconsider how you work. Some people create their own stress with their angry attitude to life which is very exhausting and stressful not only for themselves but everyone around them. The point is, try to assess where your stress comes from, and how you can make adjustments to your life. Sometimes this is hard to identify, so you might find the Life Map helpful.

Choose eight to ten prominent aspects of your life, which may include some from the above list, or you may have other aspects, and label each line with an aspect. Using the numbers as a guide, with 10 being a lot of time, and 1 or 2 being very little time, mark on the map how much you give

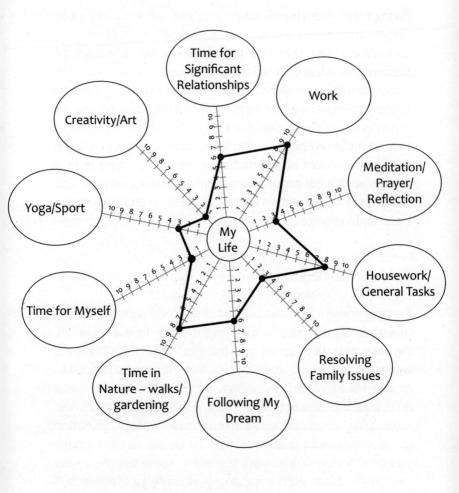

Your Life Map

to each aspect of your life. You can then join the dots to get your life map shape. The ideal is to have a balanced life, but almost everybody is bent out of shape. This map can give you a clear idea as to how you might want to adjust your energy output to bring more balance into your life.

Patterns of a lifetime

Another exercise that you might like to try is to look at patterns of a lifetime which have drained your energy. With this exercise you consider how you might adjust this pattern to bring more balance into your life, and then make a pledge to yourself to bring about a healthier change. There are almost certainly other patterns which are unique to your own life that you could add to the list. This is the absolute hub around which your entire recovery programme depends – so take your time and add to the list where appropriate.

Example:

I work long hours at the office/my desk.
Remedy: *I am going to leave my desk at 4pm each day to join a yoga and mindfulness class.*

I am always running around looking after people. I feel at the beck and call of others.
Remedy:...
....
....
....
....

I never stop until the job is finished, no matter how tired I am. I don't take a break.
Remedy:...
....
....
....
....

I am a perfectionist. I will go the extra mile to make sure everything is absolutely right.

Remedy:...
....
....
....
....

I worry that people think I am lazy.

Remedy: ....
....
....
....
....

I have to prove myself worthy.

Remedy: ....
....
....
....
....

I am a people-pleaser. I can't say "no" even when I am too tired.

Remedy ....
....
....
....
....

I always do what others want me to do rather than follow my own path.
Remedy: ....
....
....
....

I have an unhappy relationship (with friends, family, significant other, my boss) which needs to be reconsidered.
Remedy: ....
....
....
....
....

I keep going even when I am ill.
Remedy: ....
....
....
....
....

I go to bed late and get up early even though it is a struggle.
Remedy: ....
....
....
....
....

I don't take any time for myself.
Remedy: ....
....
....
....
....

I don't know how to relax, I am always busy.
Remedy: ....
....
....
....

When I am tired, I keep myself going with coffee and sugar, or I just keep going because if I stop, I will crash.
Remedy: ....
....
....
....
....

I work out at the gym but it is leaving me feeling tired rather than invigorated.
Remedy: ....
....
....
....
....

Being kind to yourself
does not have to be at
the expense of others. It
is about being respectful
towards your own needs, as
well as the needs of others,
and it teaches your children
how to respect their own
needs too.

NOTES

Chapter 2 – The Physiology of Stress

1   Baschetti R. Chronic fatigue syndrome: a form of Addison's disease. *J Intern Med*. 2000 Jun; 247(6): 737–9. doi: 10.1046/j.1365-2796.2000.00695.x.

2   Scott LV, Teh J, Reznek R, Martin A, Sohaib A, Dinan TG. Small adrenal glands in chronic fatigue syndrome: a preliminary computer tomography study. *Psychoneuroendocrinology*. 1999 Oct; 24(7): 759–68. doi: 10.1016/s0306-4530(99)00028-1

3   Tyagi A, Pugazhenthi S. Targeting insulin resistance to treat cognitive dysfunction. *Mol Neurobiol*. 2021 Jun; 58(6): 2672–91. doi: 10.1007/s12035-021-02283-3.

4   Basmaciyan L, Bon F, Paradis T, Lapaquette P, Dalle F. Candida Albicans interactions with the host: crossing the intestinal epithelial barrier". *Tissue Barriers*. 2019; 7(2): 1612–61. doi: 10.1080/21688370.2019.1612661. Epub 2019 Jun 12. PMID: 31189436; PMCID: PMC6619947.

5   Cai R, Zhou W, Jiang L, Jiang Y, Su T, Zhang C, Zhou W, Ning G, Wang W. Association between thyroid function and serum cortisol in cortisol-producing adenoma patients. *Endocrine*. 2020 Jul; 69(1): 196–203. doi: 10.1007/s12020-020-02278-5. Epub 2020 Apr 14. PMID: 32291738

6   Kaiko GE, Horvat JC, Beagley KW, Hansbro PM. Immunological decision-making: how does the immune system decide to mount a helper T-cell response? *Immunology*. 2008 Mar; 123(3): 326–38. doi: 10.1111/j.1365-2567.2007.02719.x. Epub 2007 Nov 5. PMID: 17983439; PMCID: PMC2433332.

7   Ilia J Elenkov. Glucocorticoids and the Th1/Th2 balance. *Annals of the New York Academy of Science*. 2006 Jan. doi: 10.1196/annals.1321.010

8   Skowera A, Cleare A, Blair D, Bevis L, Wessely SC, Peakman M. High levels of type 2 cytokine-producing cells in chronic fatigue syndrome.

Clin Exp Immunol. 2004 Feb; 135(2): 294–302. doi: 10.1111/j.1365-2249.2004.02354.x. PMID: 14738459; PMCID: PMC1808936.

9   Skowera A, Cleare A, Blair D, Bevis L, Wessely SC, Peakman M. High levels of type 2 cytokine-producing cells in chronic fatigue syndrome. *Clin Exp Immunol.* 2004 Feb; 135(2): 294–302. doi: 10.1111/j.1365-2249.2004.02354.x. PMID: 14738459; PMCID: PMC1808936.

10   Benhariz M, Goulet O, Salas J, Colomb V, Ricour C. Energy cost of fever in children on total parenteral nutrition. *Clin Nutr.* 1997 Oct; 16(5): 251–5. doi: 10.1016/s0261-5614(97)80037-4. PMID: 16844604.

11   Poantă L, Crăciun A, Dumitraşcu DL. Professional stress and inflammatory markers in physicians. *Rom J Intern Med.* 2010; 48(1): 57–63. PMID: 21180242.

12   Emma Kennedy, Claire L Niedzwiedz. The association of anxiety and stress-related disorders with C-reactive protein (CRP) within UK Biobank. *Brain, Behavior & Immunity - Health.* 2022; 19. doi: 10.1016/j.bbih.2021.100410.

13   Sun Y, Li L, Xie R, Wang B, Jiang K, Cao H. Stress triggers flare of inflammatory bowel disease in children and adults. *Front Pediatr.* 2019 Oct 24; 7: 432. doi: 10.3389/fped.2019.00432. PMID: 31709203; PMCID: PMC6821654.

14   Davis MC, Zautra AJ, Younger J, Motivala SJ, Attrep J, Irwin MR. Chronic stress and regulation of cellular markers of inflammation in rheumatoid arthritis: implications for fatigue. *Brain Behav Immun.* 2008 Jan; 22(1): 24–32. doi: 10.1016/j.bbi.2007.06.013. Epub 2007 Aug 15. PMID: 17706915; PMCID: PMC2211450.

15   Natarajan R, Northrop NA, Yamamoto BK. Protracted effects of chronic stress on serotonin-dependent thermoregulation. *Stress.* 2015; 18(6): 668–76. doi: 10.3109/10253890.2015.1087502. Epub 2015 Sep 28. PMID: 26414686; PMCID: PMC4893822.

16   de Souza-Talarico JN, Marin MF, Sindi S, Lupien SJ. Effects of stress hormones on the brain and cognition: evidence from normal to pathological aging. *Dement Neuropsychol.* 2011 Jan–Mar; 5(1): 8–16. doi: 10.1590/S1980-57642011DN05010003. PMID: 29213714; PMCID: PMC5619133.

17   Benjamin JJ, Kuppusamy M, Koshy T, Kalburgi Narayana M, Ramaswamy P. Cortisol and polycystic ovarian syndrome: a systematic search and meta-analysis of case-control studies. *Gynecol Endocrinol.* 2021 Nov; 37(11): 961–7. doi: 10.1080/09513590.2021.1908254. Epub 2021 Apr 5. PMID: 33818258.

18   Nepomnaschy PA, Welch KB, McConnell DS, Low BS, Strassmann BI, England BG. Cortisol levels and very early pregnancy loss in humans.

Proc Natl Acad Sci USA. 2006 Mar 7; 103(10): 3938–42. doi: 10.1073/
pnas.0511183103. Epub 2006 Feb 22. PMID: 16495411; PMCID: PMC1533790.

Chapter 3 – Balance Your Blood Sugar

1   Vitiello MV, Prinz PN, Halter JB. Sodium-restricted diet increases
nighttime plasma norepinephrine and impairs sleep patterns in man. *J
Clin Endocrinol Metab*. 1983 Mar; 56(3): 553–6. doi: 10.1210/jcem-56-3-553.
PMID: 6822653.

Chapter 4 – Deep and Restorative Sleep

1   Abbasi B, et al. The effect of magnesium supplementation on primary
insomnia in elderly: a double-blind placebo-controlled clinical trial. *J Res
Med Sci*. 2012 Dec; 17(12): 1161–9. PMID: 23853635; PMCID: PMC3703169.

Chapter 5 – Supporting Your Digestion

1   Guo C, et al. Deficient butyrate-producing capacity in the gut
microbiome is associated with bacterial network disturbances and fatigue
symptoms in ME/CFS. *Cell Host Microbe*. 2023 Feb 8; 31(2): 288–304.e8.
doi: 10.1016/j.chom.2023.01.004. PMID: 36758522; PMCID: PMC10183837.

2   Varesi A, Deumer US, Ananth S, Ricevuti G. The emerging role of gut
microbiota in myalgic encephalomyelitis/chronic fatigue syndrome (ME/
CFS): current evidence and potential therapeutic applications. *J Clin Med*.
2021 Oct 29; 10(21): 5077. doi: 10.3390/jcm10215077. PMID: 34768601;
PMCID: PMC8584653.

3   König RS, et al. The gut microbiome in myalgic encephalomyelitis
(ME)/chronic fatigue syndrome (CFS). *Front Immunol*. 2022 Jan 3; 12:
628741. doi: 10.3389/fimmu.2021.628741. Erratum in: *Front Immunol*. 2022
Mar 30;13:878196. PMID: 35046929; PMCID: PMC8761622.

4   Jiezhong Chen, Luis Vitetta. Butyrate in inflammatory bowel
disease therapy. *Gastroenterology*. 2020 Jan 14. 158(5). doi: 10.1053/j.
gastro.2019.08.064

5   Kaïs Rtibi, et al. Chemical constituents and pharmacological actions
of carob pods and leaves (Ceratonia siliqua L.) on the gastrointestinal

tract: a review. *Biomedicine & Pharmacotherapy*. 2017; 93: 522–8. https://doi: 10.1016/j.biopha.2017.06.088.

Chapter 7 – Restore Your Adrenal Glands

1   Ma C, Ma Z, Liao XL, Liu J, Fu Q, Ma S. Immunoregulatory effects of glycyrrhizic acid exerts anti-asthmatic effects via modulation of Th1/Th2 cytokines and enhancement of CD4(+)CD25(+)Foxp3+ regulatory T cells in ovalbumin-sensitized mice. *J Ethnopharmacol*. 2013 Jul 30; 148(3): 755–62. doi: 10.1016/j.jep.2013.04.021. Epub 2013 Apr 28. PMID: 23632310.

2   Liqiang Wang, Rui Yang, Bochuan Yuan, Ying Liu, Chunsheng Liu, The antiviral and antimicrobial activities of licorice, a widely-used Chinese herb. *Acta Pharmaceutica Sinica B*. 2015; 5(4): 310–15. doi: 10.1016/j.apsb.2015.05.005.

3   Diomede L, Beeg M, Gamba A, Fumagalli O, Gobbi M, Salmona M. Can antiviral activity of licorice help fight COVID-19 infection? *Biomolecules*. 2021 Jun 8; 11(6): 855. doi: 10.3390/biom11060855. PMID: 34201172; PMCID: PMC8227143.

4   Zhang RX, Li MX, Jia ZP. Rehmannia glutinosa: review of botany, chemistry and pharmacology. *J Ethnopharmacol*. 2008 May 8; 117(2): 199–214. doi: 10.1016/j.jep.2008.02.018. Epub 2008 Mar 10. PMID: 18407446.

5   Mahdi AA, Shukla KK, Ahmad MK, Rajender S, Shankhwar SN, Singh V, Dalela D. Withania somnifera improves semen quality in stress-related male fertility. *Evid Based Complement Alternat Med*. 2009 Sep 29; 2011: 576962. doi: 10.1093/ecam/nep138. Epub ahead of print. PMID: 19789214; PMCID: PMC3136684.

6   Bani S, Gautam M, Sheikh FA, Khan B, Satti NK, Suri KA, Qazi GN, Patwardhan B. Selective Th1 up-regulating activity of Withania somnifera aqueous extract in an experimental system using flow cytometry. *J Ethnopharmacol*. 2006 Aug 11; 107(1): 107–15. doi: 10.1016/j.jep.2006.02.016. Epub 2006 Apr 5. PMID: 16603328.

7   Singh M, Jayant K, Singh D, Bhutani S, Poddar NK, Chaudhary AA, Khan SU, Adnan M, Siddiqui AJ, Hassan MI, Khan FI, Lai D, Khan S. *Withania somnifera* (L.) Dunal (Ashwagandha) for the possible therapeutics and clinical management of SARS-CoV-2 infection: plant-based drug discovery and targeted therapy. *Front Cell Infect Microbiol*. 2022 Aug 15; 12: 933824. doi: 10.3389/fcimb.2022.933824. PMID: 36046742; PMCID: PMC9421373.

8   Jun J Mao, Sharon X Xie, Jarcy Zee, Irene Soeller, Qing S Li, Kenneth Rockwell, Jay D Amsterdam. Rhodiola rosea versus sertraline

for major depressive disorder: a randomized placebo-controlled trial, *Phytomedicine*. 2015; 22(3): 394–9, doi: 10.1016/j.phymed.2015.01.010.

9   Bylka W, et al. Centella asiatica in cosmetology. *Postepy Dermatol Alergol*. 2013 Feb; 30(1): 46–9. doi: 10.5114/pdia.2013.33378. Epub 2013 Feb 20. PMID: 24278045; PMCID: PMC3834700.

10   Rasangani Sabaragamuwa, et al. Centella asiatica (Gotu kola) as a neuroprotectant and its potential role in healthy ageing. *Trends in Food Science & Technology*. 2018; 79: 88–97.

11   Aboyade OM, et al. Sutherlandia frutescens: the meeting of science and traditional knowledge. *J Altern Complement Med*. 2014 Feb; 20(2): 71–6. doi: 10.1089/acm.2012.0343. Epub 2013 Jul 9.

12   Fernandes AC, et al. The antioxidant potential of Sutherlandia frutescens. *J Ethnopharmacol*. 2004 Nov; 95(1) : 1–5. doi: 10.1016/j.jep.2004.05.024. PMID: 15374599.

13   Depika Dwarka, et al. Identification of potential SARS-CoV-2 inhibitors from South African medicinal plant extracts using molecular modelling approaches. *South African Journal of Botany*. 2020; 133: 273–84, ISSN 0254-6299, doi: 10.1016/j.sajb.2020.07.035.

Chapter 8 – Post-Viral Fatigue and Long Covid

1   Ilia J Elenkov. Systemic stress-induced Th2 shift and its clinical implications. *International Review of Neurobiology*, Academic Press, 2002; 52: 163–86.

2   Assaf AM, Al-Abbassi R, Al-Binni M. Academic stress-induced changes in Th1- and Th2-cytokine response. *Saudi Pharm J*. 2017 Dec; 25(8): 1237–47. doi: 10.1016/j.jsps.2017.09.009. Epub 2017 Sep 25. PMID: 29204074; PMCID: PMC5688230.

3   Patangia DV, Anthony Ryan C, Dempsey E, Paul Ross R, Stanton C. Impact of antibiotics on the human microbiome and consequences for host health. *Microbiologyopen*. 2022 Feb; 11(1): e1260. doi: 10.1002/mbo3.1260. PMID: 35212478; PMCID: PMC8756738.

4   https://www.who.int/europe/news-room/fact-sheets/item/post-covid-19-condition

5   Yasuhito Nakatomi, et al. Neuroinflammation in patients with chronic fatigue syndrome/myalgic encephalomyelitis: an 11C-(R)-PK11195 PET study. *Journal of Nuclear Medicine*. 2014 Jun; 55(6): 945–50; DOI: 10.2967/jnumed.113.131045.

6   Tate W, Walker M, Sweetman E, Helliwell A, Peppercorn K, Edgar C, Blair A, Chatterjee A. Molecular mechanisms of neuroinflammation in

ME/CFS and Long COVID to sustain disease and promote relapses. *Front Neurol.* 2022 May 25; 13: 877772. doi: 10.3389/fneur.2022.877772. PMID: 35693009; PMCID: PMC9174654.

7   Marks DF. Converging evidence of similar symptomatology of ME/CFS and PASC indicating multisystemic dyshomeostasis. *Biomedicines.* 2023; 11: 180. doi: 10.3390/biomedicines11010180.

8   https://aonm.org/long-covid-webinar-series/

9   Pons S, Fodil S, Azoulay E, Zafrani L. The vascular endothelium: the cornerstone of organ dysfunction in severe SARS-CoV-2 infection. *Crit Care.* 2020 Jun 16; 24(1): 353. doi: 10.1186/s13054-020-03062-7. PMID: 32546188; PMCID: PMC7296907.

10   S Charfeddine, et al. Endothelial dysfunction is the key of long COVID-19 symptoms: the results of TUN-EndCOV study. *Archives of Cardiovascular Diseases Supplements.* 2022; 14(1): 126. ISSN 1878-6480. doi: 10.1016/j.acvdsp.2021.10.004.

Chapter 9 – Repair Your Mitochondria

1   Picard, Martin PhD, McEwen, Bruce S PhD. Psychological stress and mitochondria: a conceptual framework. *Psychosomatic Medicine.* 2018 Feb/Mar; 80(2): 126–40. DOI: 10.1097/PSY.0000000000000544.

2   Picard M, McEwen BS. Psychological stress and mitochondria: a systematic review. *Psychosom Med.* 2018 Feb/Mar; 80(2): 141–53. doi: 10.1097/PSY.0000000000000545.

3   Daniels TE, et al. Stress and psychiatric disorders: the role of mitochondria. *Annual Review of Clinical Psychology.* 2020; 16:1: 165–86

4   Jan-Willem Taanman. The mitochondrial genome: structure, transcription, translation and replication. *Biochimica et Biophysica Acta (BBA) – Bioenergetics.* 1999; 1410(2): 103–23. ISSN 0005-2728. doi: 10.1016/S0005-2728(98)00161-3.

5   Rahman A, Sarkar A, Yadav OP, Achari G, Slobodnik J. Potential human health risks due to environmental exposure to nano- and microplastics and knowledge gaps: a scoping review. *Sci Total Environ.* 2021 Feb 25; 757: 143872. doi: 10.1016/j.scitotenv.2020.143872. Epub 2020 Dec 3. PMID: 33310568.

6   Sun Q, Li Y, Shi L, Hussain R, Mehmood K, Tang Z, Zhang H. Heavy metals induced mitochondrial dysfunction in animals: molecular mechanism of toxicity. *Toxicology.* 2022 Mar 15; 469: 153136. doi: 10.1016/j.tox.2022.153136. Epub 2022 Feb 21. PMID: 35202761.

7   For a more comprehensive list of these medicines, see https://www.medsafe.govt.nz/profs/PUArticles/June2017/ MitochondrialDisordersMedicinestoAvoid.htm

8   Saben JL, Boudoures AL, Asghar Z, Thompson A, Drury A, Zhang W, Chi M, Cusumano A, Scheaffer S, Moley KH. Maternal metabolic syndrome programs mitochondrial dysfunction via germline changes across three generations. *Cell Rep*. 2016 Jun 28; 16(1): 1–8. doi: 10.1016/j. celrep.2016.05.065. Epub 2016 Jun 16. PMID: 27320925; PMCID: PMC4957639.

9   Nunn AVW, Guy GW, Brysch W, Bell JD. Understanding Long COVID: mitochondrial health and adaptation-old pathways, new problems. *Biomedicines*. 2022 Dec 2; 10(12): 3113. doi: 10.3390/biomedicines10123113. PMID: 36551869; PMCID: PMC9775339.

10   BC Wolverton, WL Douglas, K Bounds (September 1989). Interior landscape plants for indoor air pollution abatement (Report). NASA. NASA-TM-101766.

11   Viktorova J, et al. Native phytoremediation potential of urtica dioica for removal of PCBs and heavy metals can be improved by genetic manipulations using constitutive CaMV 35S promoter. *PLoS One*. 2016 Dec 8; 11(12): e0167927. doi: 10.1371/journal.pone.0167927. Erratum in: *PLoS One*. 2017 Oct 19; 12(10): e0187053. PMID: 27930707; PMCID: PMC5145202.

12   Zhai Q, et al. Dietary strategies for the treatment of cadmium and lead toxicity. *Nutrients*. 2015 Jan 14; 7(1): 552–71. doi: 10.3390/nu7010552. PMID: 25594439; PMCID: PMC4303853.

13   Soto-Urquieta MG, et al. Curcumin restores mitochondrial functions and decreases lipid peroxidation in liver and kidneys of diabetic db/db mice. *Biol Res*. 2014 Dec 22; 47(1): 74. doi: 10.1186/0717-6287-47-74.

14   Bagheri H, et al. Effects of curcumin on mitochondria in neurodegenerative diseases. *Biofactors*. 2020 Jan; 46(1): 5–20. doi: 10.1002/biof.1566.

15   Deng X, et al. Promotion of Mitochondrial Biogenesis via Activation of AMPK-PGC1a Signaling Pathway by Ginger (Zingiber officinale Roscoe) Extract, and Its Major Active Component 6-Gingerol. *J Food Sci*. 2019 Aug; 84(8): 2101–11. doi: 10.1111/1750-3841.14723.

Chapter 10 – Healing Herbs for Post-Viral Fatigue

1   Couzin-Frankel J. Clues to Long Covid: scientists strive to unravel what is driving disabling symptoms. *Science*. 2022 Jun 16; 376(6599).

2   Courtney E Price, George A O'Toole, The gut–lung axis in cystic fibrosis, ASM Journals, *Journal of Bacteriology*. 2021 Sep; 203(2023). doi: 10.1128/jb.00311-21.

3   Budden, et al. Emerging pathogenic links between microbiota and the gut–lung axis. *Nat Rev Microbiol*. 2017; 15: 55–63. doi: 10.1038/nrmicro.2016.142

4   Mirashrafi S, et al. The efficacy of probiotics on virus titres and antibody production in virus diseases: a systematic review on recent evidence for COVID-19 treatment. *Clin Nutr ESPEN*. 2021 Dec; 46: 1–8. doi: 10.1016/j.clnesp.2021.10.016. Epub 2021 Oct 23. PMID: 34857182; PMCID: PMC8539817.

5   Rouf R, et al. Antiviral potential of garlic (*Allium sativum*) and its organosulfur compounds: a systematic update of pre-clinical and clinical data. *Trends Food Sci Technol*. 2020 Oct; 104: 219–34. doi: 10.1016/j.tifs.2020.08.006. Epub 2020 Aug 19. PMID: 32836826; PMCID: PMC7434784.

6   Ahmadpour E, et al. Efficacy of olive leaves extract on the outcomes of hospitalized covid-19 patients: a randomized, triple-blinded clinical trial. *Explore* (NY). 2022 Oct 29: S1550-8307(22)00204-X. doi: 10.1016/j.explore.2022.10.020. Epub ahead of print. PMID: 36319585; PMCID: PMC9617633.

7   Behzadi A, et al. Antiviral potential of Melissa officinalis L.: a literature review. *Nutrition and Metabolic Insights*. 2023; 16. doi: 10.1177/11786388221146683

8   Festa J, Singh H, Hussain A, Da Boit M. Elderberries as a potential supplement to improve vascular function in a SARS-CoV-2 environment. *J Food Biochem*. 2022 Nov; 46(11): e14091. doi: 10.1111/jfbc.14091. Epub 2022 Feb 3. PMID: 35118699.

9   Jędrzejewski T, et al. COVID-19 and cancer diseases: the potential of *Coriolus versicolor* mushroom to combat global health challenges. *Int J Mol Sci*. 2023 Mar 2; 24(5): 4864. doi: 10.3390/ijms24054864. PMID: 36902290; PMCID: PMC10003402.

10   Dimopoulos TT, et al. White button mushroom (*Agaricus bisporus*) supplementation ameliorates spatial memory deficits and plaque formation in an amyloid precursor protein mouse model of Alzheimer's disease. *Brain Sci*. 2022 Oct 8; 12(10): 1364. doi: 10.3390/brainsci12101364. PMID: 36291298; PMCID: PMC9599624.

11   Singh A, Adam A, Rodriguez L, Peng BH, Wang B, Xie X, Shi PY, Homma K, Wang T. Oral supplementation with AHCC®, a standardized extract of cultured *Lentinula edodes* mycelia, enhances host resistance against SARS-CoV-2 infection. *Pathogens*. 2023 Apr 3; 12(4): 554. doi: 10.3390/pathogens12040554. PMID: 37111440; PMCID: PMC10144296.

12   Dai X, Stanilka JM, et al. Consuming lentinula edodes (shiitake) mushrooms daily improves human immunity: a randomized dietary intervention in healthy young adults. *J Am Coll Nutr.* 2015; 34(6): 478–87. doi: 10.1080/07315724.2014.950391. Epub 2015 Apr 11. PMID: 25866155.

13   Wang L, et al. The antiviral and antimicrobial activities of licorice, a widely-used Chinese herb. *Acta Pharm Sin B.* 2015 Jul; 5(4): 310–15. doi: 10.1016/j.apsb.2015.05.005. Epub 2015 Jun 17. PMID: 26579460; PMCID: PMC4629407.

14   Sagar S, et al. Bromelain inhibits SARS-CoV-2 infection via targeting ACE-2, TMPRSS2, and spike protein. *Clin Transl Med.* 2021 Feb; 11(2): e281. doi: 10.1002/ctm2.281. PMID: 33635001; PMCID: PMC7811777.

15   Metzig C, et al. Bromelain proteases reduce human platelet aggregation in vitro, adhesion to bovine endothelial cells and thrombus formation in rat vessels in vivo. *In Vivo.* 1999 Jan–Feb; 13(1): 7–12. PMID: 10218125.

16   Pekas E, et al. Combined anthocyanins and bromelain supplement improves endothelial function and skeletal muscle oxygenation status in adults: a double-blind placebo-controlled randomised crossover clinical trial. *British Journal of Nutrition.* 2021 Jan 28; 125(2): 161–71. doi:10.1017/S000711452002548

17   Messaoudi O, et al. Berries anthocyanins as potential SARS-CoV–2 inhibitors targeting the viral attachment and replication; molecular docking simulation. *Egyptian Journal of Petroleum.* 2021 Mar; 30(1): 33–43. doi: 10.1016/j.ejpe.2021.01.001. Epub 2021 Jan 21. PMCID: PMC7825908.

18   Nawrot J, et al. Medicinal herbs in the relief of neurological, cardiovascular, and respiratory symptoms after COVID-19 infection: a literature review. *Cells.* 2022 Jun 11; 11(12): 1897. doi: 10.3390/cells11121897. PMID: 35741026; PMCID: PMC9220793.

19   Wu M, et al. Roles and mechanisms of hawthorn and its extracts on atherosclerosis: a review. *Front Pharmacol.* 2020 Feb 21; 11: 118. doi: 10.3389/fphar.2020.00118. PMID: 32153414; PMCID: PMC7047282.

20   Fessler SN, Chang Y, Liu L, Johnston CS. Curcumin confers anti-inflammatory effects in adults who recovered from COVID-19 and were subsequently vaccinated: a randomized controlled trial. *Nutrients.* 2023; 15(7): 1548. doi: 10.3390/nu15071548

Chapter 11 – Healing the Brain

1   Roerink ME, et al. Interleukin-1 as a mediator of fatigue in disease: a narrative review. *J Neuroinflammation*. 2017 Jan 21; 14(1): 16. doi: 10.1186/s12974-017-0796-7. PMID: 28109186; PMCID: PMC5251329.

2   König RS, et al. The gut microbiome in myalgic encephalomyelitis (ME)/chronic fatigue syndrome (CFS). *Front Immunol*. 2022 Jan 3; 12: 628741. doi: 10.3389/fimmu.2021.628741. Erratum in: *Front Immunol*. 2022 Mar 30; 13: 878196. PMID: 35046929; PMCID: PMC8761622.

3   Safadi JM, Quinton AMG, Lennox BR, et al. Gut dysbiosis in severe mental illness and chronic fatigue: a novel trans-diagnostic construct? a systematic review and meta-analysis. *Mol Psychiatry*. 2022; 27: 141–153. doi: 10.1038/s41380-021-01032-1.

4   Verkhratsky A, Illes P, Tang Y, et al. The anti-inflammatory astrocyte revealed: the role of the microbiome in shaping brain defences. *Sig Transduct Target Ther*. 2021; 6: 150. doi: 10.1038/s41392-021-00577-5.

5   Devassy JG, Leng S, Gabbs M, Monirujjaman M, Aukema HM. Omega-3 polyunsaturated fatty acids and oxylipins in neuroinflammation and management of Alzheimer disease. *Adv Nutr*. 2016 Sep 15;7(5):905-16. doi: 10.3945/an.116.012187. PMID: 27633106; PMCID: PMC5015035.

6   Hosp JA, Dressing A, Blazhenets G, Bormann T, Rau A, Schwabenland M, Thurow J, Wagner D, Waller C, Niesen WD, Frings L, Urbach H, Prinz M, Weiller C, Schroeter N, Meyer PT. Cognitive impairment and altered cerebral glucose metabolism in the subacute stage of COVID-19. *Brain*. 2021 May 7; 144(4): 1263–76. doi: 10.1093/brain/awab009. PMID: 33822001; PMCID: PMC8083602.

7   Angeles-Agdeppa I, Nacis JS, Capanzana MV, Dayrit FM, Tanda KV. Virgin coconut oil is effective in lowering C-reactive protein levels among suspect and probable cases of COVID-19. *J Funct Foods*. 2021 Aug; 83: 104557. doi: 10.1016/j.jff.2021.104557. Epub 2021 May 24. PMID: 34055047; PMCID: PMC8142857.

8   Joshi S, Kaushik V, Gode V, Mhaskar S. Coconut oil and immunity: what do we really know about it so far? *J Assoc Physicians India*. 2020 Jul; 68(7): 67–72. PMID: 32602684.

9   De la Rubia Ortí JE, Sánchez Álvarez C, Selvi Sabater P, Bueno Cayo AM, Sancho Castillo S, Rochina MJ, Hu Yang I. Influencia del aceite de coco en enfermos de alzhéimer a nivel cognitivo [How does coconut oil affect cognitive performance in alzheimer patients?]. *Nutr Hosp*. 2017 Mar 30; 34(2): 352–6. Spanish. doi: 10.20960/nh.780. PMID: 28421789.

10   Mitsugu Yoneda, et al. Theobromine up-regulates cerebral brain-derived neurotrophic factor and facilitates motor learning in mice. *Journal of Nutritional Biochemistry*. 2017; 39: 110–16, ISSN 0955-2863, doi: 10.1016/j.jnutbio.2016.10.002.

11   Sathyapalan T, Beckett S, Rigby AS, Mellor DD, Atkin SL. High cocoa polyphenol rich chocolate may reduce the burden of the symptoms in chronic fatigue syndrome. *Nutr J*. 2010 Nov 22; 9: 55. doi: 10.1186/1475-2891-9-55. PMID: 21092175; PMCID: PMC3001690.

12   Martín MA, Goya L, de Pascual-Teresa S. Effect of cocoa and cocoa products on cognitive performance in young adults. *Nutrients*. 2020 Nov 30; 12(12): 3691. doi: 10.3390/nu12123691. PMID: 33265948; PMCID: PMC7760676.

13   Kevin Spelman, et al. Neurological activity of lion's mane (Hericium erinaceus). *Journal of Restorative Medicine*. 2017; 6: 19.

14   Saitsu Y, Nishide A, Kikushima K, Shimizu K, Ohnuki K. Improvement of cognitive functions by oral intake of Hericium erinaceus. *Biomed Res*. 2019; 40(4): 125–31. doi: 10.2220/biomedres.40.125. PMID: 31413233.

15   Roda E, De Luca F, Ratto D, Priori EC, Savino E, Bottone MG, Rossi P. Cognitive Healthy Aging in Mice: Boosting Memory by an Ergothioneine-Rich *Hericium erinaceus* Primordium Extract. *Biology*. 2023; 12: 196. doi: 10.3390/biology12020196.

16   Nagano M, Shimizu K, Kondo R, Hayashi C, Sato D, Kitagawa K, Ohnuki K. Reduction of depression and anxiety by 4 weeks Hericium erinaceus intake. *Biomed Res*. 2010 Aug; 31(4): 231–7. doi: 10.2220/biomedres.31.231. PMID: 20834180.

17   Akhondzadeh S, Noroozian M, Mohammadi M, Ohadinia S, Jamshidi AH, Khani M. Melissa officinalis extract in the treatment of patients with mild to moderate Alzheimer's disease: a double blind, randomised, placebo controlled trial. *J Neurol Neurosurg Psychiatry*. 2003 Jul; 74(7): 863–6. doi: 10.1136/jnnp.74.7.863. PMID: 12810768; PMCID: PMC1738567.

18   Borgonetti V, Pressi G, Bertaiola O, Guarnerio C, Mandrone M, Chiocchio I, Galeotti N. Attenuation of neuroinflammation in microglia cells by extracts with high content of rosmarinic acid from in vitro cultured Melissa officinalis L. cells. *J Pharm Biomed Anal*. 2022 Oct 25; 220: 114969. doi: 10.1016/j.jpba.2022.114969. Epub 2022 Jul 29. PMID: 35961210.

19   Yamamoto J, Yamada K, Naemura A, Yamashita T, Arai R. Testing various herbs for antithrombotic effect. *Nutrition*. 2005 May; 21(5): 580–7. doi: 10.1016/j.nut.2004.09.016. PMID: 15850964.

20   Moss M, Smith E, Milner M, McCready J. Acute ingestion of rosemary water: evidence of cognitive and cerebrovascular effects in

healthy adults. *Journal of Psychopharmacology*. 2018; 32(12): 1319–29. doi:10.1177/0269881118798339.

21   Moss M, Cook J, Wesnes K, Duckett P. Aromas of rosemary and lavender essential oils differentially affect cognition and mood in healthy adults. *Int J Neurosci*. 2003 Jan; 113(1) :15–38. doi: 10.1080/00207450390161903. PMID: 12690999.

22   Sehirli, Ahmet Ozer & Aykaç, Aslı & Süer, Kaya & Sayıner, Serkan. Could St John's wort have a protective effect on brain injury caused by COVID-19? *IOSR Journal of Pharmacy (IOSRPHR)*. 2021; 11: 01–03.

23   Li Y, Yang D, Gao X, et al. Ginger supplement significantly reduced length of hospital stay in individuals with COVID-19. *Nutr Metab (Lond)*. 2022; 19: 84. doi: 10.1186/s12986-022-00717-w

24   Arcusa R, Villaño D, Marhuenda J, Cano M, Cerdà B, Zafrilla P. Potential role of ginger (*Zingiber officinale* Roscoe) in the prevention of neurodegenerative diseases. *Front Nutr*. 2022 Mar 18; 9: 809621. doi: 10.3389/fnut.2022.809621. PMID: 35369082; PMCID: PMC8971783.

25   Cristina Rezende, Gustavo Vieira de Oliveira, Mônica Volino-Souza, Patrícia Castro, Juan Manuel Murias & Thiago Silveira Alvares. Turmeric root extract supplementation improves pre-frontal cortex oxygenation and blood volume in older males and females: a randomised cross-over, placebo-controlled study. *International Journal of Food Sciences and Nutrition*. 2022; 73:2: 274–83. DOI: 10.1080/09637486.2021.1972411

26   Lopresti AL. Salvia (sage): a review of its potential cognitive-enhancing and protective effects. *Drugs R D*. 2017 Mar; 17(1): 53–64. doi: 10.1007/s40268-016-0157-5. PMID: 27888449; PMCID: PMC5318325.

27   Kennedy D, Pace S, Haskell C, et al. Effects of cholinesterase inhibiting sage (*Salvia officinalis*) on mood, anxiety and performance on a psychological stressor battery. *Neuropsychopharmacol*. 2006; 31: 845–52. doi: 10.1038/sj.npp.1300907.

28   Tate W, Walker M, Sweetman E, Helliwell A, Peppercorn K, Edgar C, Blair A, Chatterjee A. Molecular mechanisms of neuroinflammation in ME/CFS and Long COVID to sustain disease and promote relapses. *Front Neurol*. 2022 May 25; 13: 877772. doi: 10.3389/fneur.2022.877772. PMID: 35693009; PMCID: PMC9174654.

29   Decker MJ, Tabassum H, Lin JMS, et al. Electroencephalographic correlates of chronic fatigue syndrome. *Behav Brain Funct*. 2009; 5: 43. doi: 10.1186/1744-9081-5-43

30   Paszkiel S, Dobrakowski P, Łysiak A. The impact of different sounds on stress level in the context of EEG, cardiac measures and subjective stress level: a pilot study. *Brain Sci*. 2020 Oct 13; 10(10): 728. doi: 10.3390/brainsci10100728. PMID: 33066109; PMCID: PMC7601981.

31   Sokal P, Sokal K. The neuromodulative role of earthing. *Med Hypotheses*. 2011 Nov; 77(5): 824–6. doi: 10.1016/j.mehy.2011.07.046. PMID: 21856083

32   Oschman JL. Perspective: assume a spherical cow: the role of free or mobile electrons in bodywork, energetic and movement therapies. *J Bodyw Mov Ther*. 2008 Jan; 12(1): 40-57. doi: 10.1016/j.jbmt.2007.08.002. Epub 2007 Dec 3. PMID: 19083655.

33   Chevalier G, Sinatra ST, Oschman JL, Sokal K, Sokal P. Earthing: health implications of reconnecting the human body to the Earth's surface electrons. *J Environ Public Health*. 2012; 2012: 291541. doi: 10.1155/2012/291541. Epub 2012 Jan 12. PMID: 22291721; PMCID: PMC3265077.

Chapter 12 – Stress, Pain and the Endocannabinoid System

1   de Melo Reis RA, Isaac AR, Freitas HR, de Almeida MM, Schuck PF, Ferreira GC, Andrade-da-Costa BLDS, Trevenzoli IH. Quality of life and a surveillant endocannabinoid system. *Front Neurosci*. 2021 Oct 28; 15: 747229. doi: 10.3389/fnins.2021.747229. PMID: 34776851; PMCID: PMC8581450.

2   Crocq MA. History of cannabis and the endocannabinoid system. *Dialogues Clin Neurosci*. 2020 Sep; 22(3): 223–8. doi: 10.31887/DCNS.2020.22.3/mcrocq. PMID: 33162765; PMCID: PMC7605027.

3   Lutz B, Marsicano G, Maldonado R, Hillard CJ. The endocannabinoid system in guarding against fear, anxiety and stress. *Nat Rev Neurosci*. 2015 Dec; 16(12): 705–18. doi: 10.1038/nrn4036. PMID: 26585799; PMCID: PMC5871913.

4   Maldonado R, Cabañero D, Martín-García E. The endocannabinoid system in modulating fear, anxiety, and stress. *Dialogues Clin Neurosci*. 2020 Sep; 22(3): 229–39. doi: 10.31887/DCNS.2020.22.3/rmaldonado. PMID: 33162766; PMCID: PMC7605023.

5   Neumeister A, Seidel J, Ragen BJ, Pietrzak RH. Translational evidence for a role of endocannabinoids in the etiology and treatment of posttraumatic stress disorder. *Psychoneuroendocrinology*. 2015 Jan; 51: 577–84. doi: 10.1016/j.psyneuen.2014.10.012. Epub 2014 Oct 22. PMID: 25456347; PMCID: PMC4268027.

6   Maldonado R, Cabañero D, Martín-García E. The endocannabinoid system in modulating fear, anxiety, and stress. *Dialogues Clin Neurosci*. 2020 Sep; 22(3): 229–39. doi: 10.31887/DCNS.2020.22.3/rmaldonado. PMID: 33162766; PMCID: PMC7605023.

7   Russo EB. Clinical endocannabinoid deficiency reconsidered: current research supports the theory in migraine, fibromyalgia, irritable bowel, and other treatment-resistant syndromes. *Cannabis Cannabinoid Res.* 2016 Jul 1; 1(1): 154–65. doi: 10.1089/can.2016.0009. PMID: 28861491; PMCID: PMC5576607.

8   Russo EB. Clinical endocannabinoid deficiency reconsidered: current research supports the theory in migraine, fibromyalgia, irritable bowel, and other treatment-resistant syndromes. *Cannabis Cannabinoid Res.* 2016 Jul 1; 1(1): 154–65. doi: 10.1089/can.2016.0009. PMID: 28861491; PMCID: PMC5576607.

9   Bosch-Bouju C, Layé S. Dietary omega-6/omega-3 and endocannabinoids: implications for brain health and diseases [internet]. *Cannabinoids in Health and Disease.* InTech; 2016. doi: 10.5772/62498

10   Neil R. Smalheiser. A neglected link between the psychoactive effects of dietary ingredients and consciousness-altering drugs. *Front. Psychiatry.* 2019; 10: 291. doi: 10.3389/fpsyt.2019.00591.

11   Gertsch J. Cannabimimetic phytochemicals in the diet: an evolutionary link to food selection and metabolic stress adaptation? *Br J Pharmacol.* 2017 Jun; 174(11): 1464–83. doi: 10.1111/bph.13676. Epub 2017 Jan 16. PMID: 27891602; PMCID: PMC5429335.

12   Neil R. Smalheiser. A neglected link between the psychoactive effects of dietary ingredients and consciousness-altering drugs. *Front. Psychiatry.* 2019; 10: 291. doi: 10.3389/fpsyt.2019.00591.

13   Fede C, et al. Sensitivity of the fasciae to the endocannabinoid system: production of hyaluronan-rich vesicles and potential peripheral effects of cannabinoids in fascial tissue. *Int J Mol Sci.* 2020 Apr 22; 21(8): 2936. doi: 10.3390/ijms21082936. PMID: 32331297; PMCID: PMC7216169.

14   Johnson SA, Rodriguez D, Allred K. A systematic review of essential oils and the endocannabinoid system: a connection worthy of further exploration. *Evid Based Complement Alternat Med.* 2020 May 15; 2020: 8035301. doi: 10.1155/2020/8035301. PMID: 32508955; PMCID: PMC7246407.

INDEX

Note: page numbers in *italics* refer to information contained within tables.